OCTOPUS
ON A
TREADMILL

GIFTY ENRIGHT

*This book is dedicated to Dada,
for making me feel I deserve to be loved just
by virtue of being alive.*

FOREWORD
By Joanna Lumley, OBE

All working mothers have had that moment, when we catch a glimpse of ourselves in the hall mirror, on a Tuesday morning at 7.45am; over stuffed school bag in one hand, shopping list poking out of our hip pocket, polishing our work shoes on the back of our trouser leg, notes for our important meeting smeared with marmalade clutched under our arm, a haunted look in the left eye, hair metaphorically (and sometimes literally) standing on end and screaming 'Get a bloody move on!' to some hapless child or partner. In the unlikely event that we have time, we may pause to ask ourselves, 'What happened to me?' before soldiering on with our day like an octopus on a treadmill.

I remember many such moments as I juggled raising my son with my marriage, my career and home life – while still trying to hang on to my reason. That is why I have so much respect and admiration for mothers who work outside the home.

In the 80s, we read the articles in the glossy magazines about 'women who had it all' – the big job, the perfect family and enough time to hit the gym every day so that they looked absolutely fabulous to boot. Then came the 'yummy mummies' who had to forever look like they never had children. The very thought makes me tired! The truth is that we were never designed – physically, emotionally or spiritually – to withstand the frenetic and impossible demands that modern life and society put upon working mothers. We are only human, something will always give; and more often than not, it is our health and wellbeing.

It seems to me that people who should know better often suggest that the multiple challenges working mothers face can be solved with a pill or a hormone patch. There is a place for all that, of course, but few seem to be looking holistically at the root cause of the stresses and strains we face.

We are thinking, feeling, sophisticated and beautiful multifunctional creations. What we feed ourselves physically, emotionally and spiritually has a real effect on our ability not just to keep going, but to flourish and blossom again and again throughout the many wonderful stages of our lives. We must remember to love and nourish ourselves, and perhaps relearn how to do so.

Gifty Enright's wonderful book encapsulates the timeless truth that what a woman puts into her body, mind and spirit can either weigh her down or buoy her up to live a better, stronger, healthier and happier life.

Gifty has gently woven science, wisdom, humour, experiences from her life and the lessons from different cultures; creating a book that is easy to read, practical and an eye-opening reminder of how and why we need to live a better life.

The glib (perhaps male) onlooker might say that living a good life as a busy working mother is not rocket science. Well I, like many others, might reply, 'No, it's much more complex than that.'

Octopus on a Treadmill provides insights that will chime with the experiences of so many women who have had that 7.45am 'haunted' moment. However, this book is also like the moment that follows on the best of days, when you open the front door and the sun suddenly begins to shine, and you know that this is going to be a good day.

Every working mother needs to read this book, if for nothing else, to know that you are not alone and to have a good laugh, as it is hilarious in parts. I wish I'd had this book when I was starting out – it is a celebration of all women.

"To call woman the weaker sex is a libel;
it is man's injustice to woman.
If by strength is meant brute strength, then,
indeed, is woman less brute than man.
If by strength is meant moral power,
then woman is immeasurably man's superior.
Has she not greater intuition,
is she not more self-sacrificing,
has she not greater powers of endurance,
has she not greater courage?
Without her, man could not be.
If nonviolence is the law of our being,
the future is with woman.
Who can make a more effective appeal to the heart
than woman?"

~ Mahatma Gandhi

Contents

PART ONE

BARKING UP THE WRONG TREE

CHAPTER ONE

WHOSE LIFE IS IT ANYWAY?

God couldn't be everywhere so he created mothers.

~ JEWISH PROVERB

'How are you, Gifty?' the doctor asked.

His question was well meaning, but it left me confused. Why was he asking me how I was? I had brought my baby to his surgery for a routine check-up. My mother was in tow to enquire about another age-related ailment or other. *I* wasn't on the agenda.

OK, there was, of course, that small matter of me having recently undergone double major surgery: one procedure to remove my appendix and the other to go into my abdomen to explore why it had become completely distended with fluid. And, did I mention, I had also given birth naturally, with no painkillers – not even pethidine – just a few days before the surgery?

I had always been one of those people who would rather sleep off a headache than take medicine. I lived a healthy lifestyle, didn't overindulge in anything in particular and this was my second child. The pregnancy had been straightforward enough for me to be allowed a home birth. Now, before you start thinking I am some hessian-weaving, sandal-sporting hippy because I opted for a home birth, I want to assure you that this isn't the case. I just wanted to have my baby in the natural surroundings of my home, without a man in a white coat bearing down on me and telling me which position to adopt for the delivery. Plus, with a home birth, I got to have two midwives in attendance throughout and didn't have to fight with other pregnant women for their attention. If you have had a baby in an NHS hospital, you will understand where I am coming from. There seems to be a perpetual shortage of midwives. Yep, there was a method to my madness.

The birth was actually idyllic. I went into labour at 6am, in a birthing pool in my kitchen, and by noon it was all done and dusted. The most stressful thing was my husband trying to toast crumpets for the midwives halfway through my contractions. I had my mum in attendance as well. My sister was halfway to the shops with my 5-year-old son – who had to be distracted from Mummy screaming – when she got the phone call to come back because the baby had arrived.

An hour later, I had been cleaned up and was tucked up in bed with my son in the cot beside me while I had a nap. The following day, I was up and about and cooking as if nothing dramatic had happened. I was also completely oblivious to the fact my life was about to be turned on its head.

Two days after the birth, I was struck down with diarrhoea. After 12 hours of turning myself inside out, we called the doctor who came to see me at the house. He took one look at me and phoned for an ambulance. For my sins, the ambulance driver didn't know the area very well (this was before the invention of satellite navigation, and yes, I am that old) and spent half her time asking which way to turn. This obviously did not instil me with confidence. For that 30-minute ride to the hospital, I felt every bump in the road and, frankly, I could have done without feeling like I was going round in circles, as the driver asked for directions from her colleague, who was in the back with me. It also didn't help that after a few hours of being poked and prodded by doctors at the first hospital, it was decided that I needed to be transferred elsewhere, as they didn't have the expertise to treat me. That meant yet another ambulance ride, but mercifully the driver knew where he was going this time, so the bumps in the road didn't feel so bad.

At the second hospital, there was the matter of whether I should be admitted to the maternity or the surgical ward, as they still weren't sure what was wrong with me. At this point appendicitis was ruled out, but as well as the diarrhoea, I didn't seem to be responding to the intravenous antibiotics I'd been given.

Eventually, after a day or so of more tests, the decision was made to cut me open and find out what was wrong. While they were in there, they took out the appendix, as it was slightly inflamed and they didn't want to take the risk of going back in there if it later turned out to be the culprit after all. Due to the amount of antibiotics I had been given, whatever was causing the infection in my abdomen in the first place had already died by the time they operated, so the doctors couldn't establish the cause of it. All they could do was drain my abdomen and put me back in the recovery ward.

Morphine is a good thing, and I can completely understand why people get addicted to it. Not only did it take away my pain, but I also had the dubious gift of hallucinations. These took the form of full-blown conversations about my innards with a bearded consultant in a white coat. My husband later informed me that none of the consultants matched that description. What can I say? The consultant of my hallucinations was very attentive and had intimate knowledge of inner workings. And this was very comforting.

When I finally came to properly and was transferred back to the maternity ward with tubes everywhere, my mother brought in my baby, as naturally every new mother wants to cuddle their baby. I had to resign myself to staring down at the poor sleeping child. I couldn't hold him because of the tubes. There was also the small matter of my sore breasts, which were fighting their way through the web of apparatus. I didn't want to disappoint my mother, but the whole breastfeeding thing had become a bit of an endeavour.

Let me digress here and talk about the sore breasts some more. My milk had come in before I was whisked away in the not-so-luxurious ambulance. Being a dutiful mother who intended to breastfeed for two years, which was then The World Health Organisation's (WHO) recommendation, there was no way I was going to allow my milk to dry up. (The pressure we mothers put ourselves under is simply insane.) I got hold of one of those electric breast pumps and while the doctors were deliberating about what was wrong with me, I pumped away on schedule. I was going to breastfeed if it killed me! Give me a recommendation, and I will stick to it like glue.

Thank God for the distraction of expressing breast milk, because I was completely oblivious to the fact that my poor husband was at his wits' end. He would go home whenever he got the chance and cry his eyes out, as he was convinced I was going to die. His mother, who came as soon as she heard I was in hospital, later told me about the weeping. Unbeknown to me in my breast pumping, Earth Mother-mode, I was getting weaker and it was touch and go whether I was going to survive. The surgery was just to drain my abdomen of the fluid build-up and see if there was anything else in there causing it. All anyone could do was hope for the best.

Don't you just love it that after all the advances in medicine and technology within the developed world, sometimes it still gets to the point where we are reduced down to pure, old-fashioned hope? Thankfully, the diarrhoea had stopped by this stage so my poor husband stopped having to change me all the time. I didn't like the nurses doing this because they weren't gentle enough. I had a bit of a tear down below from giving birth and the nurses seemed to ignore this, which caused me a lot of discomfort. So I reserved this important job for my husband. (I am not entirely sure whether this was an added factor to his crying – despite the 'for better or worse' vow, no one quite signs up for that!) Anyway, his expert changing skills meant he amassed a bit of a following with the nurses, so there was an upside.

The surgery worked and the fluid didn't return. But with three things to recover from (the surgeries to remove my appendix and the fluid build-up, plus giving birth), the morphine proved a godsend. The hallucinations were a small price to pay. I had a catheter too – such bliss! I didn't have to get up for anything; weeing just took care of itself. I for one would buy myself a portable catheter any day. I drink two litres of water a day, which comes with a lot of weeing, and I also have a phobia of public toilets. There must be a gap in the market for a portable, everyday use catheter that you can wear under your suit.

When my husband recovered from the fact that I wasn't going to die, the surgery had been a success and the fluid wasn't going to return, we discovered that my milk had dried up. After all that expressing to establish the supply (if that doesn't make you feel like a dairy cow, nothing will), my body decided that double surgery plus childbirth was enough trauma for anyone to cope with. No amount of expressing would coax a drop of milk out. Luckily, I'd had enough of expressing anyway, and at least it meant one less body part to manipulate on top of everything else I had to cope with. I was happy to kick the Earth Mother to the kerb for a while in order to focus on my survival, and survival it was. The doctors had begun to reduce my morphine dosage, so the pain was kicking in. Without the drug, the friendly, reassuring consultant that only I could see disappeared too. I was left with the real ones, whose body language said it was about time I went home and stopped wasting their time with my mystery infection. Plus, this is the NHS so no one gets to hog a bed – there is a waiting list.

As soon as the tubes were taken out and I was up and eating horrid hospital food, I was sent on my merry way with a bunch of painkillers, some antibiotics and a bewildered look in my eye that posed the question, 'What just happened here?'

Once back home, I had to set my alarm for an hour before my normal rising time to take my painkillers. This numbed the pain enough so I could go to the toilet. I soon established my routine and after another couple of days of the baby tugging at my empty breasts (don't ask me why he did this, but both of us found it comforting and besides, I was hardly in a position to fight anyone), my milk surprisingly came back in. I was back to breastfeeding as if I had never been away. Nature truly is amazing and there is nothing like a recommendation from the WHO to keep a conformist like me plugging away at an empty breast!

The road back to recovery was torturous and I was on painkillers for longer than I care to remember. My doctor urged me to come off them, but couldn't provide any alternatives to dealing with the pain. I always received a vague reply when I asked why I was still hurting and was reminded that I'd had three things happen to me in quick succession, and that I had to be patient and give my body time to heal.

I had my mother to help me deal with the daily grind of looking after two small children, but she was no spring chicken and had her own health challenges to deal with. Each of her journeys up and down the stairs carried their own drama. My sister popped in at least once a week to do the housework and although my husband was an absolute star throughout all of this, he still had to go to work. He did his best to keep everything together without going to pieces himself.

It was Benjamin Franklin who said that nothing is certain except death and taxes. This couldn't have been more true than when I found myself confronting my annual tax return while still on painkillers, and not having earned any income for a while. Life has a way of going on regardless of what is actually going on. The bills keep on coming despite the other dramas unfolding. When your world is falling apart, the tyranny of normality and the mundane can bring you to your knees.

So, when the doctor asked me how I was, it was like being roused from a deep sleep. He held my gaze while I got my head around the fact that someone was asking about me. He persisted and asked, 'How are you recovering from the surgery?' once again.

He was perfectly within his rights to enquire about my wellbeing. The disturbing thing about this was that after everything I had been through, he had to remind me that I was actually recovering from surgery. This shows you the pecking order in which we women put our self-care, and also the extraordinary responsibility that we carry as primary carers.

How did we end up here, lugging the burden of the world on our shoulders? Caring for children, our home, our husbands, our ageing parents, not to mention holding down a job?

It all used to be nicely defined within gender-mapped roles. The women stayed at home and looked after the children and the men went out to work. Then the economy and our lifestyles started to change. One income, in some cases, wasn't enough anymore.

Additionally, women got it into their heads that whatever a man could do, they could do as well. We started venturing into the workplace. What we didn't bargain for, though, was that nothing was going to change on the home front and that we would still remain the primary carer regardless of how demanding our jobs were. So here we were. Men carried on doing what they had always done, but the poor old women had to multitask just to run to a standstill.

For the women who didn't go out to work, life became infinitely more complicated. It was no longer just about doing the chores, cooking dinner and putting on a bit of lippy before the hubby came home; they now required a PhD just to manage the endless emails from school, not to mention the dentist and doctor appointments. It seems like every child these days is allergic or has to see a consultant for something or other. Did I mention play dates, sleepovers and school-gate politics?

Life has got infinitely more complicated. Women, for some bizarre reason, decided to do more. Our parents decided to have the temerity to live longer and now we're all in a pickle and everyone is stressed out. You can't have a decent conversation with someone for more than three minutes without their eyes darting to their phone in response to some notification. This is at a time when what we need the most is to create sustaining relationships that will help us to combat stress and feel connected.

In an article in *The Huffington Post* concerning research from Medco Health Solutions, a pharmacy-benefit manager in the US, from 2001 to 2010, 25% of women (one in four) received medication for a mental health condition, compared to just 15% of men. Antidepressant use among women has gone up 29% since 2001. The report also showed how, in 2010, anti-anxiety medications were used by 11% of women. This was almost twice the rate seen among men (5.7%).

There are similar figures for the UK as well. A study by the women's campaign group, Platform 51, showed that 30% of the women they surveyed were taking antidepressants. The upshot is that on both sides of the pond, one in three women are on antidepressants. Now, why is this and why are the figures halved when it comes to men?

How did we women end up medicating ourselves just to be able to cope? And what effect is all this medication having on our biology? Are we living the lives that suit us? Could, perhaps, our lives be back to front? Why are we so stressed out? Does anyone live the good life anymore? What are men doing that we aren't? Are we biting off more than we can chew? Are we allowing the men in our lives to do their fair share?

Women are battling on multiple fronts: childcare, career, marriage and ageing parents, and yet most of the time we lack the skills to deal with these battles when they are raging. Then there are the typically female issues, such as:

- Lack of confidence.

- Self-image (does my bum look big in this? By the way, why the hell do we even have to ask?!)

- Minimising our achievements and watching less capable men beat their chests to the promotions that are rightfully ours.

- Failing to step up to a challenge because we are waiting for someone to give us permission or pat us on the back.

Let me digress here, as this is a personal bugbear of mine. The way women underestimate their talents and skills drives me to distraction. As far as I'm concerned, every business owner with half a brain should employ a mother. The flexibility she may not always be able to offer will be more than made up for by the skills that she will bring. When you employ a mother, you get 10 for the price of one. That makes good business sense, as it goes straight to your bottom line.

You get pregnant, have a baby, come back to work after your maternity leave and it's like you've been living on Venus for the past six months. So, your priorities are different because you are raising (and let's not be dramatic here) another human being! You might want to change your hours around a bit, but that doesn't mean you can't focus on a presentation or lead a team. We all know you need the skills of a UN negotiator to broker peace between warring toddlers and simultaneously manage the plumber who insists on showing you his builder's bum every time he goes under the kitchen sink. Somehow those same people skills are minimised the moment you get to the office. There is a 'situation' between two members of your team that requires your peacekeeping skills. You also have to deal with the chauvinistic additional employee that has been added to your team. He doesn't have to report directly to you and lets you know it at every turn. You haven't quite worked out which bit of the matrix he fits into, or indeed how you got caught up in the matrix in the first place, but you are saddled with him and his rotten attitude. Due to the vagaries of the matrix management, you still have to manage him. Please tell me you see the parallels with the warring toddlers and the plumber? Before you start saying 'I don't have the skills to handle this' - listen up. You have been doing this all along in your kitchen without batting an eye. The difference here is just geography.

It might be a little difficult for people to maintain eye contact with you when you are talking about next year's objectives with wet patches around your nipples because you didn't express on schedule. Your nipple pads may not have been built for this kind of volume of milk, but once the said nipple pads have been changed, the patches have dried out and you have given yourself a talking to about sticking to your expressing schedule, there is no reason why the conversation about next year's objectives cannot be resumed without you feeling like there has been a loss of respect and credibility. As Eleanor Roosevelt said: 'No one can make you feel inferior without your consent.' The fact that you can produce breast milk, feed another human being and have a business conversation (hopefully not all at the same time) in my book gives you more than enough credibility. Think about it. Men will only have to deal with the business conversation, yet we surrender our power to them all the time.

Let me tell you about my sister-in-law. She was a director at a multinational company and was heading for the stars. As some women are wont to do at some stage in their lives, she decided to try for a baby. After a few years of trying she got pregnant with triplets. She was, of course, over the moon. In the early days she didn't mention the pregnancy at work. Then, in the middle of a meeting one day, she felt unwell, went to the ladies' and realised she was bleeding. Every pregnant woman knows that bleeding, especially in the first trimester of a pregnancy, isn't a good thing. She cleaned herself, finished the meeting and then went to seek medical help. What dog-eat-dog world do we live in that makes a woman feel she has to carry on a meeting in the middle of a miscarriage, so as not to be seen as weak by the boys? Imagine the mental toughness it takes to be able to carry on, business as usual, in the middle of a miscarriage?

This story has a happy ending. While she sadly lost one of the triplets, she went on to carry the twins to full term and she's subsequently given birth to two more children.

Luckily, the corporate world is changing and it's perhaps not as brutal towards women as it used to be. We can now work from home and some employers have very flexible working patterns for women, which allows them to work around their children. That said, women have a responsibility to accelerate and manage this change in attitude. No one wants to be militant about women's issues in the workplace and get marginalised, but we owe it to ourselves to inform our male colleagues of the challenges that we face wherever possible. We have to drag our husbands and partners with us into this change as well, and we need to show our daughters how strong they are and educate them about their talents and value to society. We need to teach them not to underestimate themselves or wait for someone to give them permission to go after what they want. If they do, they will be waiting for a long time.

That was a long digression, so back to women battling on several fronts. We are battling, but we are more than equipped to deal with the fight. I come from a long line of strong women. I was never allowed to forget that my great-great grandmother, Yaa Asantewaa, was the warrior queen of the Ashanti Kingdom in Ghana who took on the British in 1900. (More about her exploits in Chapter 16.) So, although I never doubted my capability as a woman, I too got lost in the myriad challenges of modern life and forgot which way was up.

Stick with me and in the following chapters I will show you exactly how I found my way and how you too can rock your life with your innate talent as a woman. We are blessed, as women, to be beautifully complex. We can focus on our strengths and biology (yes, that's right, our biology, hormones and all) to live the life that is right for us, allows us to thrive and makes our hearts sing. This kind of existence will give us the courage to look life squarely in the eye and say, 'Bring it on.'

CHAPTER TWO

LIFE IS BACK TO FRONT

*Man sacrifices his health in order to make money. Then he sacrifices
his money to recuperate his health. Then he is so anxious about his
future that he does not enjoy the present; the result being that he
does not live in the present or the future. He lives as if he is never
going to die, then dies, having never really lived.*

~ DALAI LAMA

There was a generation of women who thought that whatever a man could do, a woman could do better. If you were one of them, and I certainly was, you had complete disdain for the women of the earlier generation who sat at home and expected their husbands to take care of them financially. You were going to take the corporate world by storm. But, before you knew it, you were a high-flying executive in a big house complete with electric gates, children and a nanny. You needed something to take the edge off because you found your own life disconcerting. You never paused to think whether this was the life you wanted. You bought into the dream of a shiny new car, a big house in suburbia and 2.4 kids. But then you started losing your religion because nothing made sense anymore. All you knew for a fact was that you were constantly knackered, stressed out, resentful and felt menopausal all the time, even though you were nowhere near 50!!!

You are probably nothing like me, but humour me as I take you through what I did. I went to school and did what I had to do. Then I went to college, studied hard, specialised in accountancy without even knowing why apart from to make my parents proud, and before I knew it I was an accountant and thinking 'what the hell??!'

I soldiered on, read a few self-help books and decided I was going to do something for myself, so I branched into IT. With my eyeballs still revolving in my head as I wondered where my life was going, I then decided to do what really made my heart sing and trained as a life coach. Back then, life coaching was still very much in its nascent stages and very much derided. It was certainly not a profession that people recognised. People told me to get a grip. How could I go from accountancy, an old-fashioned, established profession, to life coaching? Anyway, despite what other people thought, I loved it, excelled at the training and passed with flying colours, only to realise that building your own business is no picnic. For starters, there is the dreaded marketing, which, to the initiated, is a dark art. I soon retreated back into the cocoon of the safe corporate world and back into IT, where you get paid every month and, so long as you do a good job and keep your head down, you can do just fine. Meanwhile, something inside of me was slowly dying. I was making money and ticking all the boxes but there was an undercurrent of disquiet.

Hold on a minute, here comes a distraction. Luckily, I got married along the way. I felt I had messed about long enough and it was about time I produced an offspring. Out pops said offspring and life as I knew it was subsumed by nappies, sick, mother and baby groups and a vague sense that I was being left behind, which only added to the disquiet I previously felt.

I eventually got back to work, but my heart wasn't in it because now my priorities were different and my life felt infinitely more complex. Someone needed me and made me feel appreciated, but they were not in the position to give me a bonus or a promotion, or even pay me for that matter. The contribution a new being can make to your life and sense of self is minimised by society because it is not hard currency. I still wanted to be the kick-arse whatever, but now I had to work harder and smarter and plan a lot more. Every now and then my colleagues thought I was distracted because I had dropped one of my multiple balls. Were they projecting? Let's give them the benefit of the doubt. I was not going to give them the satisfaction.

I owed it to my mother's generation to make it to the top in the business world. 'Whatever a man can do, a woman can do better,' was my mantra, as I carried on pushing myself. Sometimes it was like treading treacle. I was constantly exhausted, but I had to have it all and I was damned if I was going to be the one who let the side down.

My son came home one day asking for a sibling. Apparently, everyone in his class had one and he felt left out. I was nothing if not competitive, so I jumped on my poor, unsuspecting husband and hey presto, junior number two was en route.

Soon I was back in the twilight zone with a new baby and the accompanying nappies, sick and everything in between. The sleepless nights killed me. It was much harder this time round because I was older. I couldn't remember it being this gruelling, but I am a trooper so I soldiered on.

Back to work after maternity leave, and I encountered more of the same. I felt envious of my male colleagues. They didn't have to live a whole lifetime before 9am every morning. Worse still, I had to compete with them on the work front. Women have fought for a level playing field in the workplace, so now here we are, but someone please tell me how this field can in any way be level?

Even with the most involved husbands (I mean the wiping-your-backside-when-you're-ill type of involved), we still somehow end up doing more. So when we take on the working mother role, too, are we making a rod for our own backs? Have we scored an own goal? And are we too busy 'having it all' to realise this? Even when the roles are reversed and the man is the primary carer, how many times will a woman come home from work and just put her dainty feet up in front of the TV and expect to do nothing but be fed and watered? We come home and switch roles with the man without even batting an eye. The man heads down to the pub with his mates because he has been with the kids all day and we are back to where we started. This is stereotypical, of course, but you get my drift.

Whichever way we cut it, one way or another we end up burnt out and reaching for the antidepressants or alcohol, or, in some cases, both. We have to take the edge off somehow. If you continually have to take the edge off your life, you are not living the right life for you. You can go on in that vein for a while but your body has a way of letting you know that it has had enough.

I think we live our lives back to front. We go for the trappings of what we think we want, rather than what we actually want. Unfortunately, we may only realise that the things we thought would make us happy haven't had the desired effect until we have spent years chasing them. It would be great if after we left college we were given a list that said: 'These are the things that will make you happy.' Unfortunately, there is no such list and we have to figure them out for ourselves. Society complicates this quest by giving us the wrong pointers. Everyone sucks up to the one with the big job, the money, the big house, the perfect kids, etc., so we think that is what we have to go after. We set out to create the life that will give us those things with no regard for our own values, strengths and our raison d'etre. We somehow leap to the conclusion that the things other people have and look up to will make us happy too.

Life is about balance. You have to discover your values and find what makes you tick and causes your heart to sing. Then you need to go after it for a living. A lot of us don't ever work this out. We just respond to life rather than deciding on the life we want to live. This may be down to societal pressure or even our parents' dreams. We go after things that we are not even sure we want, but we have to keep up with the Joneses. Yes, we have to earn a living and we can't all sit by a camp fire with flowers in our hair singing *Kumbaya*, but we can live a life of balance and focus on what is truly important to us, how we can best contribute to our society as women and how to live the life that suits and supports us. If we don't, we will be needing the pills or the wine to take the edge off the tyranny of our life.

CHAPTER THREE

A MAN'S STORY

This is a man's world, this is a man's world.
But it wouldn't be nothing, nothing without a woman or a girl.

~ JAMES BROWN, *IT'S A MAN'S MAN'S MAN'S WORLD*

For the past decade, the M25 motorway has played a significant role in my life. I work as an IT consultant around the Heathrow area for a multinational company. I live in Hertfordshire and although the journey from home to the office is only 35 miles, it can take up to an hour and a half, depending on when I hit the motorway. I routinely spend around three hours a day during the week on it, and it's where much of my personal growth has taken place. One day, I was merrily pootling along listening to the radio when I heard a man being interviewed about being a single 'mother'! That got my attention. I immediately thought, 'This is a man doing a typically female role. I wonder how that is going for him'. You see, sometimes you have to step outside yourself and look at things with a different lens to be able to appreciate what being a woman is all about. Another reason why this got my attention was because I knew the journalist who was interviewing him. She had been the MC at an event I organised. So I contacted her and she put me in touch with the producers who reached out to the man on my behalf. Luckily, he was happy for me to interview him. I contacted him for a chat and he was such a hoot. I, of course, approached him with my preconceptions about a man being in a woman's world and having an easy ride. I must say, I had a few surprises and some of my expectations were sharply managed. Andy is a single father of three children, aged 18, 12 and seven. The youngest was just two when unfortunately Andy's ex-wife decided that she did not want to continue their relationship. He was, of course, devastated. Initially, their two youngest went to live with Andy's ex-wife, but after a relatively small amount of time she agreed that they were better off living with him and she moved away. That is how he became his children's primary carer.

As a working 'mother', he was certainly in at the deep end. Below is our chat. Enjoy.

GE: What is your philosophy on life?

Andy: Life is a series of challenges, and it's about surviving these challenges.

GE: What does success mean to you?

Andy: Success in life is being the best that I can be by living. I try to achieve this by growing, developing, learning and loving, taking risks and facing challenges.

GE: What makes a successful parent?

Andy: Knowing your children and wanting them to be the best they can be.

GE: How have you been able to get your priorities straight with regards to the children?

Andy: Making a lot of mistakes and learning from them.

GE: How have you managed juggling work and childcare?

Andy: By choosing work that fits around my children. Spending time with them is very important to me.

GE: What are the advantages and disadvantages of being a man in this role?

Andy: Women are naturally good at networking with each other. Being a man, there is a lot of pressure to be the breadwinner and much status, power and authority is attached to this. I struggled with letting go and fell off a cliff with that one.

I also had to make sure that my children had adequate contact with other women, including my sisters, mum, my friends and their mother.

I think as a man I've got to constantly fight not to become isolated. That's hard and some of the other difficulties concern getting over to both men and women that I'm not a victim. I chose this, it's not something that was forced upon me and it's not something I'm trying to escape. I'm embracing it.

The advantages are that I have escaped the pressure that is heaped on women because I am not seen as a mum. I am not subject to the same judgment. I'm a white, able-bodied, heterosexual male and I know that I naturally have advantages in society as a result of this.

GE: How did you cope at mother and toddler groups, being around women only?

Andy: It was hard and I did feel like an outsider. Some of the women were suspicious of me, but the bottom line is that everyone wants to talk about their children.

GE: It's taken for granted that the woman will be the primary carer, but when a man takes on this role it has a halo effect. What do you think about this?

Andy: My experience has been that people think 'this shouldn't happen', so they want to fix me. They see it as a situation that they need to change. I find this quite bizarre and also incredibly frustrating at times.

GE: What sacrifices have you had to make?

Andy: I don't think sacrifice is the right word, but I have had to make compromises regarding money and status in return for time with my children.

The other big compromises have been sex, a good relationship and more time for me.

GE: Really? Is the visual of a man with a pushchair in the park having women leaping from the bushes and throwing themselves at him a myth then?

Andy: I can sort this one out straightaway. You don't want those sorts of women. You want someone who wants you for you rather than for your relationship with your children.

GE: What else do you think you had to compromise on?

Andy: I think another compromise is that I don't meet the people I used to. My social circle now revolves around the children.

On the money side, I wish I didn't have to make that compromise and I could mark my children's rites of passage, such as throwing a big 18th birthday party for my son, etc., but we do other things instead that don't cost a lot of money.

GE: What were the rewards of choosing to put your children first?

Andy: I really, really do know my children. I have to say this three or four times before people normally hear it. Choosing to prioritise the time with them has been a privilege and the things I've found out about them has often blown me away. I have lived many lives and travelled a lot, but I feel incredibly lucky to have been able to fully experience my children growing up and to play a big part in moulding their lives.

Another advantage, after I got through the initial struggles of being their primary carer, was that there was a quiet inner peace. The satisfaction I felt when I went through something with my children and knew that they were safe and that they were inspired really touched something in me. I don't experience that with anything else.

My relationships with my wider family also improved. I have four sisters – two older and two younger – and a mum. We have always been a close family, but our relationship was taken to a deeper level and I gained their friendship just by the sheer amount of time we spent together with the children.

GE: Were any of these rewards unexpected?

Andy: The inner peace. I used to be such a worrier. I also used to be quite loud and charismatic. People now describe me as a quiet, thoughtful and patient person.

GE: What's been harder than you thought it would be?

Andy: Coping with my pride and not having much money. Also multitasking and keeping on top of everything was quite difficult.

Initially, putting everybody else first was hard, because this can make you lose yourself a little bit. You forget who you are. Sometimes I did disappear down a hole. You also have to keep on going for your children. That was hard.

GE: Did you at any point feel that life was passing you by?

Andy: Oh crikey! Yes, I remember thinking I was old and the best was behind me. I did, however, manage to keep what was really important and that was: caring and nurturing my children.

GE: How did you keep on top of everything and did you at any point question your choice?

Andy: For a long time I didn't keep on top of everything. I used to beat myself up something chronic over it and then I finally got to a place of figuring out what was most important and focusing on that. I can't stress enough how hard this was.

I learned to allow myself to cry. I used to use sad films to set me off. I also used to call certain friends and family and just say: 'Look, I just need to come round because I need to cry.' They would just let me sob and then I'd go off and I'd be fine.

I was terrible. I did everything for my kids and others and didn't leave any time for myself. I had to learn to find time for me, otherwise I was no good to anyone.

When it comes to the traditional roles that males and females play, the males are the providers and protectors and the females are the nurturers. I think those roles need to intertwine, otherwise both genders suffer.

GE: Did you at any point question your choice?

Andy: No, I don't think I did. I constantly questioned how I was with the kids, but every parent does that.

GE: Did you consider another model of paying somebody else to look after your children whilst you continued with your career?

Andy: I would never do that.

GE: Steady, you know I work full-time, right?

Andy: I just couldn't. I might get myself in trouble here, but I don't understand that. Why would I place that much importance on making money? I would love to make more money, don't get me wrong, but it's just not at that cost.

GE: Some people don't have a choice because of financial pressures.

Andy: And I do, and I think it is a personal choice, and it's also a hard one.

GE: What do you wish someone had pulled you aside and told you when you first became a primary carer?

Andy: 'Trust yourself.' Each time I've gone through something difficult it's been hard, but I've also learnt something.

'Andy, let people help you,' would have also been a good piece of advice.

I'd also like to have heard, 'Don't feel so isolated.'

Your children challenge you to be the best person you can be and so what I actually say to young couples is to first spend time deciding what sort of family they want to be. I tell them to think about what's important to them: their beliefs, their resources, what they're striving for and what comes where in the pecking order.

I don't normally give advice. If I think someone is struggling, I try and give them time rather than advice.

GE: Do you think you made the right choice?

Andy: Absolutely, 100%.

GE: My last question: What would you change if you could go back and do it all again?

Andy: Nothing. Genuinely. There were some really difficult times, but I don't know what I would have missed out on learning if I hadn't gone through them.

I also think spending your life thinking 'I should have done this' or 'I should have done that' is a waste of time.

There you have it, a man's point of view. Hopefully, that should give us some inspiration to stop beating ourselves up. We are all in the same boat. The job we do as women is phenomenal. In the following chapters, I will go through how you can get your priorities straight and not fall off a cliff, as that is always a danger.

THE ROAD TO DAMASCUS

No one saves us but ourselves. No one can and no one may.
We ourselves must walk the path.

~ BUDDHA

I went to see my GP with my list of 14 symptoms. I kid you not. I'd put them on a spreadsheet so I could track when I started getting better. That is why I know the number. Here they are because I know you will want to know:

	Symptoms
1	Night sweats
2	Achy joints
3	Foggy brain
4	Memory issues
5	Heart palpitations
6	Sore breasts
7	Anxiety/mood swings
8	Headaches
9	No libido
10	Heavy periods
11	Irregular periods

12	Urinary infections
13	Digestive issues
14	Extreme tiredness

Table 1. My Symptoms

As usual with the NHS, you have to literally walk into the doctor's surgery holding your uterus in your hand to be taken seriously. After a couple of appointments, where I felt I was getting nowhere because I was being told that my symptoms were consistent with my age, blah, blah, blah, I decided to take my life in my own hands (aka, succumb to pressure from my husband) and go private.

Picture this: Here I am following my consultation with one of the leading gynaecologists in Harley Street, walking towards Great Portland Street tube station in London, completely stunned out of my wits, clutching HRT at the grand old age of 44. How did this happen? Did I mention I was only 44? It might seem old to some, but the recognised age for the start of the menopause in the UK is 50. OK, so you can be perimenopausal for up to 15 years before your actual menopause, but I wasn't one of these 'special' women. I was a normal, run-of-the-mill mother with no major medical issues to speak of. In the consultant's waiting room, I spied a couple of other older women trying desperately to hang onto their youth. You know the type: too much makeup, expensive clothes and more money than sense. They were going to defy the ageing process if it killed them. That was not me. I was in the prime of my life. Wasn't life supposed to begin at 40? Well, I was only four years into that, so what was I doing clutching HR fucking T? For starters, I didn't do drugs and that included painkillers. I had hessian-weaving tendencies and preferred to sleep a headache away rather than take drugs. How was I going to cope with a long-term prescription of hormone replacement therapy comprising tablets and creams? Also, did I mention that I am lactose intolerant? Do you know that a lot of tablets have lactose in them? For years I used to wonder why I would have a headache, take a tablet and end up with a bad stomach, so I decided to stay off tablets altogether, as I just couldn't be bothered anymore. That is how I ended up snoozing headaches away. So, a long-term prescription of tablets to manage my hormones until the menopause was a non-starter for me.

To add insult to injury, I had a scan and the consultant was surprised that my bone density was less than ideal. Apart from the fact that my eyeballs were revolving in my head by the unwelcome reality that I was facing, I was now being told that there was something wrong with my bone density. By the time I got back to Great Portland Street tube station, I'd developed a limp.

I'd been fine that morning. OK, I had 14 different symptoms, but I sure as hell wasn't limping. What was the matter with my right hip now? How did I end up here? This was simply insane. The doctor had smeared some hormone gel on my arms just to show me how to apply it and I was convinced that when I got back to the office I was suddenly going to jump the first man that crossed my path because I'd be overcome by this sudden influx of hormones. In spite of this, I had to chair a meeting, business as usual, as if I hadn't just been told my hormones had decided to go on strike without telling me.

That was when I knew something had to give. I just couldn't continue the life I was living. I was trying to have it all, but it was costing me my health. My high achieving – trying to tick the boxes that society required me to tick – was robbing me of my bone density at 44. Life had to change. If I'm honest, I had been suffering from my symptoms for at least four years before I plucked up the courage to go and see a consultant.

It has been a long journey from those 14 symptoms. I have learnt a lot along the way and I continue to learn, because I am a nerd like that. People marvel at my age when I tell them how old I am. It's been a hard-won fight on several fronts. My hope is that I can pass on the lessons I have learnt so that you don't one day find yourself standing by a tube station questioning your bone density and your sanity.

What do we really need in order to live a happy and balanced life?

Maslow's hierarchy of needs is a theory that was proposed by the American psychologist Abraham Maslow in 1943. To this day, it remains a very popular and widely accepted framework for human behaviour.

Maslow's hierarchy is used to describe the pattern of human motivation. So, in the diagram below, people will normally start off looking to fulfil their basic physiological needs, such as food, shelter and clothing, before moving up and eventually ending up at self-actualisation.

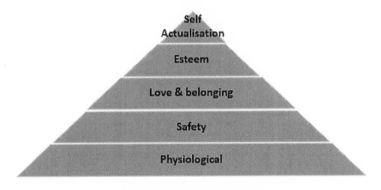

Figure 1. Maslow's Pyramid

In the subsequent chapters, we will work our way around the pyramid and I'll map Maslow onto the holistic way of living.

I intend to take you through the following aspects of life, which draw certain parallels with Maslow's model. I'll explain what we should be doing in the following aspects of life in order to ensure we live a balanced one:

- Physical
- Emotional
- Mental

- Spiritual

This is a holistic approach. You can't take care of one part and ignore the others without suffering in some way or another.

If I had my way, I would start with the spiritual, but I don't want to lose half of you before we get past the starting blocks. The word spiritual has all sorts of connotations that can turn a lot of people off, which I think is a real shame. I promise you that I'm not a holy roller. To me, spirituality is the philosophy that colours the lens through which life can be viewed. It can be used to make sense of a lot of things that can seem confounding. In Maslow's hierarchy, it is up there with self-actualisation and self-transcendence.

I believe that spirituality has an effect on your thoughts, which in turn impacts the mental plane on which you operate. Thoughts affect your emotions, which then impact your physical being. That is why wellbeing is a holistic endeavour. Therefore, this is another pyramid I will be exploring, which I will call the Life Pyramid:

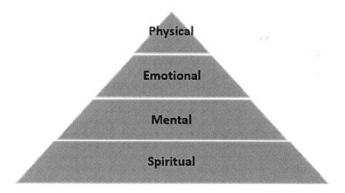

Figure 2. Life Pyramid

This is sort of upside down to Maslow's hierarchy, where you start with the spiritual and work your way up to the physical, but the two ideas are not diametrically opposed. I will expand on this further in Chapter 14.

Then there is the chakra system, which is popular in Hindu, Buddhist and Jain philosophy. In my view, it mirrors Maslow's beliefs. There are seven chakras:

1. Root
2. Sacral
3. Solar Plexus
4. Heart
5. Throat
6. Third Eye
7. Crown

I could do another pyramid, but I think you have had enough of pyramids by now. The main point to note with the chakras, however, is that the first one is positioned at the root where the genitals are. You work your way up from there. If you stick with me, we'll go into this more in the spiritual section of the book. Here, we'll see how everything is exquisitely interwoven. It's sheer elegance.

The point of this book is to take you through a holistic and balanced way of living, where your goals and your actions are aligned to your purpose, and therefore your life. This means you are not living your life against yourself and you are not leaving any part of yourself uncared for. If you live this way, you will not age prematurely or reach for any form of stimulant or antidepressant, and your hair will not fall out because of stress. You will become aware of what is important to you and prioritise your life around that, treating yourself as the precious commodity that you are.

If you live this way, you'll beat the frazzle and will be able to look life courageously in the eye and say, 'show me what you've got!'

PART TWO

FIRING ON ALL CYLINDERS

CHAPTER FOUR

THE EXQUISITE INTELLIGENCE
OF THE FEMALE BIOLOGY

If women ran the world we wouldn't have wars,
just intense negotiations every 28 days.

~ ROBIN WILLIAMS

When it comes to the female body, the only word I love to use is 'exquisite'. It has two meanings, both of which are applicable:

» Extremely beautiful and delicate

» Intensely felt

Maybe I'm biased because I'm a woman, but that is how I see myself on all levels. Notice the meanings don't include the words 'pretty', 'stunning' or 'gorgeous'. You can be beautiful without fitting these descriptions. It may be a cliché, but beauty radiates from within and I subscribe to that. Women are intrinsically beautiful. We need to recognise our femininity and manage it accordingly. We are beautiful and we are strong and delicate at the same time. We also feel things intensely.

There are many things about the female form that have captivated artists for millennia. Haute couture celebrates the female form. This is on the physical side of things, but I am going to focus on female biology; the menstrual cycle to be precise. This is what drives feminine energy and ancient cultures have long recognised this. The Apache Indian tribe plus several African tribes, including the

Dogon and Ashanti, have special rituals around menstruation. In our industrialised age and through our pursuit of women's rights, we have unfortunately thrown the baby out with the bath water. Some women feel that in order to be recognised, they have to hide their femininity under a bushel and come across as masculine. What is that about? Why can't you go toe-to-toe with a man in a well-cut shift dress and power heels? It may be distracting for the man, but that is his problem to manage, as you are there to talk business. Don't get me wrong, I do the trouser suits too, probably more than the dresses, as our weather will only allow all of two days a year in which to bare our legs. The point is: you should not be hiding your light under a bushel. What you are wearing should be appropriate for the occasion, but in all manner of seriousness, how long did it take for this conversation to degenerate into what a woman is wearing rather than what she has got to say? Let's go on to what I have got to say. Our bodies are an asset to us. Implicit in our menstrual cycle is both a physical and an emotional navigation system. Ignore it at your peril. You have to know how it works and honour its rhythms in order to live the life that suits you. You don't want to live a man's life; they have different hormones and a different navigation system to follow. So when we discount our feminine power and decide to become masculine, we create conflict and pay a heavy price for it.

As a woman, you cannot perform at the same level throughout the month. Your biology simply won't let you. This is not a weakness, it's a strength. So what do we do? We cancel out the biology with pills so that we can feel the same throughout the month. This is simply insane. It is the equivalent of cancelling the seasons and having summer throughout the year. How long will it take before the hosepipe ban is put in place? What will happen to all the different fruits and vegetables we grow throughout the seasons? What will happen to all the beautiful autumn colours? Apart from stripping our lives of the rich tapestry of variation in emotions, our natural rhythms and the way we feel physically, we will lose our feminine essence. Not only that, we will become unhinged. We were created this way for a reason. The ancient cultures were onto something when women were put in moon huts together when they were menstruating. It had nothing to do with being unclean, although that is the obvious conclusion people leap to. It was to give the women time to put themselves back together. Spiritual traditions put a lot of emphasis on menstruation days. This is because women are so pivotal to societies in the roles that they play. I will, in later chapters, prove to you the effect the emotional wellbeing of women has on the general population as a whole. This is why they should be supported to keep them emotionally balanced at all times. The ancient cultures knew this. There is a Native American Indian saying, which goes, 'The fastest way to destroy a tribe is to first destroy the moon lodge.' (The moon lodge being where the women lived while menstruating.) There is research now to support this, as I will go on to prove.

Let's look at the menstrual cycle and what happens during each phase. We'll do this by taking a quick dip into GCSE biology. Back in the day, my biology lesson about the female reproductive system was a cringefest. My fellow pupils and I wanted the ground to open up and swallow us, and this was at an all girls' school! The teacher, also female, did her best to gloss over everything and no one was invited to ask any questions. The lesson was all over in a flash. Where was the celebration of the magic of the female in that? Or the wonder about the cycle that brings life into this world? Perhaps if we had been taught to celebrate our bodies, I would not have found myself, some 30 years later, limping to a tube station in a state of total shock and clutching HRT!!! Anyway, here goes the biology lesson.

Below are the four main phases of the menstrual cycle and the hormones at play:

Phase 1 Menstruation

Days 1-4. Bleeding occurs. The lining of the uterus disintegrates and is shed. This is due to low levels of progesterone.

Phase 2 Follicular Phase

Days 4-14. The uterine lining that was shed in the bleeding phase grows back. This is due to high levels of oestrogen. Follicle-stimulating hormone, or FSH, is also secreted, stimulating the production of follicles in the ovaries, which contain eggs.

Phase 3 Ovulation

Day 14. The egg (called an ovum) is released from the ovaries into the fallopian tubes for fertilisation. This is due to LH (luteinising hormone). Oestrogen is also present in significant quantities around the time of ovulation, and it can interact with other hormones to increase libido.

Phase 4 Luteal Phase

Days 14-28. After ovulation, the empty follicle that once contained the egg begins to secrete the hormone progesterone to thicken the lining of the uterus and prepare it for the possible implantation of an embryo.

If the egg is not fertilised, then we are back to Phase 1 and the cycle continues.

Implication of the Phases

Now we know the science, let's map it onto life and see how we can make the best of our biology and how it makes us feel. I have put everything on the diagram over the page to try and give you a visual link between biology and your actions.

The follicular and ovulation phase is your happy time of the month. The first four days of your period can be rough, especially if you are bleeding heavily, but it is also a release. You may feel a bit tired in the first week due to the blood loss. This first week of the cycle is when you are supposed to be taking things easy, with the emphasis on nurturing yourself and releasing what doesn't serve you. Treat yourself to a massage or pedicure, have a haircut and go for gentle walks. This is not the time for full-on gym sessions. Read the book that has been languishing on your Kindle for ages waiting for attention rather than choosing to host a sleepover for the kids. If there is any party going on, it should be a pyjama party for you and close friends, with everyone bringing their own food. This is not the time to give of yourself, rather it is the time to take and to allow your loved ones to support you. You have to learn to be good to yourself in that sense. If you allow yourself to take one week in the month for yourself, it will put you in a far better position to give and nurture for the following three weeks. When we get to communication skills later on, you will be equipped to ask for space for yourself during this phase, without anyone feeling threatened. This is your winter so you have to learn to chill out.

Menstrual Cycle

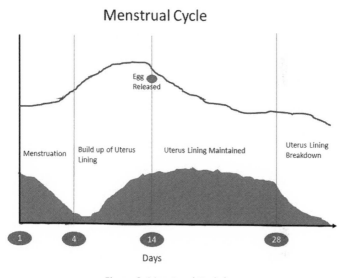

Figure 3. Menstrual Cycle*

In around week two, you move into what is the equivalent of spring. Your bleeding has stopped and everything seems fresh. If you have taken good care of yourself in your winter, then you should feel rejuvenated and you will normally be full of the joys of spring. Everything is brighter, you'll see new beginnings everywhere, and you'll feel positive, ambitious and want to take on the world. This is when you are beginning to feel fertile, sensual, bold, dynamic and energetic. You'll be naturally flirtatious and you are more likely to buy clothes, makeup and other items to help yourself feel more attractive. Your body is getting ready to release an egg for fertilisation. Your

*Image sourced from BBC GCSE Bitesize

oestrogen levels are high and this will make insulin more effective, which in turn will stimulate the production of testosterone, the hormone that regulates the sex drive. This is nature's way of signalling to women to have more sex, as they are at their most fertile. This is when you should be scheduling your date nights, shopping trips with your girlfriends and starting new projects, etc.

When you enter your Luteal Phase from week three, you are still on a high. You are now in your summer. This is when you build on the things you started in your spring. You are ripe and you feel able to nourish, nurture and focus on others. You feel receptive and better equipped to make sacrifices. This is when your kids think you are the best mum in the world, your sisters love you and your friends know you are in their corner. You feel creative and abundant and can give of yourself freely. Your communication skills are heightened. This is the time to give the presentation that will blow your boss and colleagues away. It's also a good time to work on relationships and have difficult conversations. You are in a giving mode and can handle criticism without flying off the handle. You can even have a productive conversation with the builder.

However, the second half of the Luteal Phase can be problematic for some women. This is the week before your next period; your autumn. The American College of Obstetricians and Gynaecologists estimate that 85% of women experience at least one symptom related to premenstrual syndrome per month. Progesterone, which is on the increase in this phase, helps the body make cortisol, and this is normally higher in people with raised stress levels. This helps to explain why you might feel a bit moody and wired. If you are already stressed out due to life in general, or you're not managing your previous phases properly, then this phase will exacerbate the problem. This is the time when you tend to look for comfort in sugary foods. I used to go through umpteen packets of wine gums. There was always a stash in my handbag that would go untouched until I hit this phase. Then I would suddenly start stuffing my face.

Listed over the page are some of the symptoms associated with this phase:

Emotional

- Deep sadness or despair

- Irritability

- Feelings of tension or anxiety

- Mood swings

- Crying

- Disinterest in daily activities and relationships

- Trouble thinking or focusing

- Feeling out of control or overwhelmed

Physical

- Fatigue

- Loss of libido

- Food cravings or binge eating

- Sore breasts

- Feeling bloated

- Headaches

In my case, I used to barricade myself in the bedroom at weekends and my kids and husband would only come in if they fancied a stab in the eye! They would resort to communication by text. Until I hit this phase, I was a calm and measured person. Then I would turn into Bertha Mason from Mr Rochester's attic in *Jane Eyre*, complete with mad hair. At no point did anyone point out to me that this was a red flag for something amiss with my hormones, and that it could be managed with a change in lifestyle.

This is your autumn, so it should be a time for introspection. By all means barricade yourself in a room if you need space, but the

OCTOPUS ON A TREADMILL

stab in the eye should be optional! You will be feeling intolerant so it's perhaps not the time to confront the builder, as you might find yourself changing contractors halfway through the loft conversion. You will feel like tidying up a lot as you'll be craving order during this phase to ease the sense of overwhelm that you are feeling. This is the time to do the tax return that you have been procrastinating about. You are at your most intuitive and those of you who meditate (more on this in Chapter 14) will be able to go deeper. You may begin to withdraw from social situations as well, and that is OK too. You may not be feeling your most energetic, but don't let the exercise slide. Working out releases endorphins that make you feel good about yourself and goodness knows, during this phase you'll need this boost the most. If you are ever going to feel fat and dissatisfied with your body, this is the time when those feelings will come to the fore. As well as tackling the tax return, why not take on the housework and give everything a deep clean? Pick up your rug and whack the bejesus out of it. It will feel good. This is your moment to alphabetise the contents of the grocery cupboard or face the filing head on. You are feeling this way because you are at a crossroad; you are either pregnant or about to shed the lining of the uterus and have your period. Either way, something is about to go down, hence the heightened sense of disquiet. Work with your body. We get all the cues from nature, but if we don't listen to them or if we medicate them away, the wires get crossed and before we know it we've turned into hormonal bitches that no one wants to be around.

These signals are there to guide us and give us nudges when we are out of balance. They are not there to overwhelm us enough to stab someone in the eye. When things get that bad, there is something terribly wrong. It means your life is not aligned to your feminine cycle, which means you are not aligned with your purpose. No woman can get away with this for long. This is why it is rather worrying when we are forced to medicate our feminine energy away. We do this because we don't embrace our cycles and live around them. Instead we see them as an inconvenience. Our periods are sometimes called the 'curse' and other derogatory terms. In the Akan cultures in Ghana, they have big celebrations when a girl has her first period. She is encouraged to dress up and her passage to womanhood is broadcast to all. Sumptuous food is prepared for her and she is made to feel special. These cultures understand the pivotal role that the woman plays in society and they celebrate it. Just handing a girl a packet of tampons or a bag of sanitary towels and talking about the hygienic aspect of things, as we do in the West, is not enough. Someone needs to explain the emotional impact and what happens during each phase, as well as what the girl can do to support herself. We might not want to go back to consigning menstruating women to moon huts, but we can allow them to have the same rituals the huts afforded them, which is about taking the pressure off. They need to be in a supportive environment and to be allowed to carry on with their own self-care.

The lifestyle changes that I will be exploring in subsequent chapters should equip you to handle these changes better. The food, hydration, exercise and emotional management will go a long way towards allowing you to live a better life around your cycles.

There is intelligence in the way our bodies work and embracing and working with that intelligence is the only sustainable way forward.

CHAPTER SIX

WHAT IS YOUR FUEL?

Let food be thy medicine and medicine be thy food.

~ HIPPOCRATES

Physical Part 1: Nutrition

The word physical covers our basic needs, such as air, food, water, shelter and clothing. These needs have to be met in order for us to function. A problem arises when the shelter has to be a certain square footage on a particular street complete with electric gates, just so that we can feel we have arrived. The sacrifices we make from the shift of fulfilling a basic need to being the envy of our friends is never worth it. To live a life that meets our higher purpose and leaves us fulfilled, we have to know where the boundaries are between basic need and the extraneous. We also have to be aware of the opportunity cost of going out to work at a job we hate, just so we can live in a certain square footage with three en suite bathrooms and a sauna that is never used! When you look logically at the way most of us live, it's simply insane. Know your needs, meet them, and after that your choices should be about the opportunity cost. Is the choice at the cost of your joy? Is an 18-hour day at the office really worth the cost of having no friends or having the sort of friends who are attracted to you because of what you have rather than who you are?

The physical is about taking care of your physical body and your physical environment. These include:

- Food
- Shelter/transport
- Self-care

Food

I am going to start with food because a lot of women have a diabolical relationship with it. Some have been on one type of weight loss diet or another since they were teenagers. The pressure we are under to look a certain way is unbelievable. If you happen to be a woman working in the corporate world, then you'll be no stranger to the fact that the way you look is the invisible point in your performance appraisal plan. We all know that women at the top look a certain way. We're all aware there is a 'newsreader' type of look. It is unwritten, it is unspoken, but it is there. The corporate-woman-look. Then there is the 'I-have-always-got-to-look-nice-for-my-husband-look', not to mention the 'what-will-the-neighbours-think-look'. None of these looks pays homage to the 'I-am-a-woman-who-is-comfortable-in-my-skin-and-I-am-just-going-to-dress-the-way-that-works-best-for-me-look.' Due to pressure to look a certain way, for one reason or another, there is always some diet fad holding us to ransom and it is truly never ending. How about just eating to feel good in your body and look the way you are happy to look? The fact is, some people have no idea how they are happy to look. Their look has been dictated for so long by something outside of themselves that it is really difficult to make the decision: 'I am going to eat for me.'

When it comes to food, I subscribe to Hippocrates, who said, *'Let food be thy medicine and medicine be thy food.'*

I believe food should serve multiple purposes:

- Look good
- Taste good

- Have healing properties (i.e. it does good inside you, rather than just occupying space and coming out!)

- Satisfy hunger

A lot of people eat for all sorts of reasons other than hunger. They may be bored, upset or even just reacting to the food being right in front of them. Some people eat constantly, so they don't even know what hunger feels like. If you are eating for the wrong reasons, more often than not you won't be eating the right stuff. If you eat the right thing at the right time, you'll be surprised by the amount of rubbish you will cut out and how you will lose weight without even trying. This is because the body regulates itself. I am not just saying this…I am speaking from experience. If you eat well, your body will fall to its natural weight level. The problem is, a lot of women aren't happy with their natural weight because they are subscribing to some airbrushed, unattainable model. They then adopt unhealthy eating practices to reach their preferred level. But no airbrushed image is attainable. Even if you delude yourself into thinking you have attained it, you will soon find that it is unsustainable. Then, before you know it, you are beating yourself up, staring at a tub of ice cream and feeling like a failure. How can you break this cycle?

It's easy – and I mean easy – to break this cycle. Be realistic, eat the right food and you will not crave crap. I have done this myself, but to be fair, I've never been someone who was content to eat crap. I have always had relatively good eating habits, or so I thought before I found myself limping towards a London tube station. (No, I don't think I will ever get over that, and there will be a few more references to the said tube station before this book is over, so you better brace yourself for it.)

I have always enjoyed a good diet. Well, I did within what I knew about nutrition. Then suddenly I found myself suffering from hormone imbalance issues at 44. I had a choice. Go on HRT forever, with all its associated risks, or find an alternative. I decided to find an alternative. I tried a lot of things, including consuming only the right foods for my dosha (the doshas in Ayurveda express unique blends of physical, emotional and mental characteristics), taking herbs that smelt like rotten eggs and sticking lotions and potions up my vagina to draw the heat out of my body. I guess this had something to do with the hot flushes I was experiencing. Last but not least, I had tubes shoved up my rectum. AKA colonic irrigation.

Indulge me here while I detour into the colonic irrigation saga. I promise I will not be gross. It started off well enough when I felt this lovely warm sensation and smelt the scent of lavender wafting around. Afterwards, though, I thought I could just go and sit on the loo and let nature take its course, but I was told to hold it in for as long as I could. That is how I found myself on the train from East Croydon to St Albans with my butt cheeks clenched and an other-worldly expression on my face. (The journey takes a little over an hour on the fast train.) I daren't cough or sneeze lest I ended up sitting in a warm, brown puddle. Throughout the journey, I debated how to arrange my face so no one would guess the battle raging in my intestines. In order to survive this ordeal, I called my best friend who happens to live in San Francisco. I talked her through the absurdity of the situation and tasked her with taking my mind off the aforementioned battle. People in San Francisco are supposed to be out there, so I knew she could handle it. In case you are wondering, I survived the train journey with no mishaps, but I almost caved in during the additional 20-minute drive to my house. There is something about being on your own that makes you feel that social norms can 'go take a jump'. Anyway, I got home and made a beeline for the bathroom, where the lavender-fragranced contents of my bowel were disposed of in a suitably civilised manner. By the way, I am telling you all this to hopefully save you from a similar ordeal on a train journey. If you start eating well now you will save your hormones from going crazy from years of abuse. The irony of this is that it is coming from someone who thought she ate well.

What did I learn from trying all these therapies? Well, you have to change your mindset about food and eat for health rather than for weight loss, or, for that matter, anything else. If you eat for health, you'll be more patient with yourself if the weight doesn't drop off in 24 hours. The good thing about eating for health, though, is that you will lose the weight as a by-product and you'll normalise to your correct body weight. The body is designed to get rid of toxins and anything that doesn't serve it, but it needs to be properly supported in order for it to operate efficiently. Eating for health ensures that you are giving the body the correct fuel that it needs to operate. This is just the same as a petrol car failing to work if you put diesel in it. Your body will need to try harder to use the crap you put into it. Then it will finally pack up one day, when you are least expecting it.

I love knowing what I am eating and what it will do for my body once it's ingested. I refuse to use my body as a dustbin to hoover up crap that I will have to work very hard to get rid of later. I am just lazy like that. I work out for health rather than weight loss and do the absolute minimum that I can get away with. Think of it this way. Do you want your body to use the energy it has to get rid of toxins? Or do you want it to use it for maintenance and health-giving duties? The choice is yours.

Food for health

When it comes to food, eat wholefoods and cut out the processed crap as much as you can. You'll see a significant change in your body, and your life for that matter. Even though I thought I ate well – i.e. I wasn't bingeing on ice cream and crisps – I still had a lot to learn about eating for health. Luckily, I am lactose intolerant, so that put paid to most desserts and there is only so much fruit salad you can eat before you start hating fruit of any shape. This also meant I wasn't over doing it on the sugar either. But I was eating lots of red meat. One of the many things I had to do on the path to health was keep a food diary. When I realised how much red meat I was consuming a week I was staggered.

Below was a typical week's dinner menu:

- Monday: Spaghetti bolognaise

- Tuesday: Chilli con carne with white rice.

- Wednesday: Pork chops with vegetables and potatoes.

- Thursday: Chicken in tomato sauce with white rice.

- Friday was junk food day so anything went. I can't have pizza because of the cheese but it would normally be some sort of takeaway. Chinese, Indian or fish and chips.

- Saturday: Grilled fish with potatoes or white rice and vegetables.

- Sunday: Roast. This was normally lamb, but sometimes it was steak with potatoes and vegetables.

Apart from Fridays, I cooked every day. By cooking, I don't mean heating stuff up in the microwave. I was, however, skipping breakfast most days or having a breakfast bar on the go. Lunch was whatever I could lay my hands on in the canteen at work, but I must say I do love a hot lunch so no doubt there was more meat involved. I wasn't eating between meals or stuffing my face with crisps, biscuits or chocolate. As far as I was concerned, I should have been getting an A* for my diet, but my body was telling me otherwise. Why was this? Why was I always tired? Why were my hormones playing up? Why did I have a list of 14 symptoms…actually it was 15 now, if you add the bone density issue. (OK, my imaginary limp had long since disappeared, so I will stick to the 14 for now.) Also, why had I suddenly developed sugar cravings around certain times of the month? This was especially odd, as I didn't even have a sweet tooth. Hopefully, you know what phase of my cycle I am referring to here. Why did I have problems with my digestion and sometimes suffered from bloating when I had been nowhere near dairy? Why did I get easily constipated? Why did I find myself retaining water on a business trip to Singapore?

A further digression. I was lying by the pool soaking up the sun in Singapore, as one is wont to do in sunny climes, when the hotel masseuse approached me. Never one to pass up on a massage, I plumped for some reflexology. The Singaporean masseuse, an elderly man with kind eyes, spent a few minutes faffing around with my foot before looking at me and declaring I was retaining water. What the hell I was supposed to do with that piece of information was beyond me. Can't a woman just relax by the pool for once during her hard-won time away from the family without being delivered some death blow or other? On top of that, I'd brought all sorts of weird herbs and potions into the country in the name of Ayurveda, in order to balance my hormones. For all I knew, I could have been languishing in some prison cell for bringing the said herbs and looking for a human rights lawyer to come and rescue me, just like Bridget Jones. Anyway, I told the kindly masseuse that I would go and see my doctor as soon as I got back home.

The thing is, if you sit in front of your doctor with your list of symptoms, they won't enquire what you are eating and whether you are eating right. They'll just look for the drug that they know will deal with the symptoms. The side effects are just the cross you have to bear. Sometimes, if you are really lucky, you will be given extra drugs for the side effects as well. To be fair to the medical profession (I have to be nice here as my very close friend is a doctor. If I'm not, the kids won't be allowed over to her house for a sleepover. Then what will I do in my winter when I need a break from the children to take care of myself?), in the allotted 10 NHS-minutes, you couldn't really go into people's diet and lifestyle even if you wanted to. That is not what current medicine is about, well, not on the NHS anyway. If you want to look at the problem holistically, that is, from the cause to how you can deal with it, without being dependent on a drug for the rest of your life, you'll have to do it yourself. You will have to go and see different specialists and piece the jigsaw together. With my 14 symptoms, that would have meant a lifetime spent seeing specialists.

On the subject of the use of prescription drugs, in the US in 2004, a group of researchers (Gary Null, PhD, Carolyn Dean MD, ND, Martin Feldman, MD, Debora Rasio, MD and Dorothy Smith, PhD) published a paper called 'Death by Medicine'. One of the staggering findings was that conventional medicine caused an estimated

783,936 deaths a year in the US, making it the leading cause of death –12% higher than heart disease and 42% higher than cancer. The deaths were caused by things such as adverse reactions to drugs, medical errors, infections, unnecessary procedures and surgery-related issues, to name a few.

I am not trying to scare you off going to your doctor. What I am trying to do is explain that like so many things in life, prevention is better than cure. Eat for health and save yourself from becoming a statistic.

Back to what I was eating during a typical week. What was wrong with it exactly? Let's do some troubleshooting. The problem was that I was eating way too much red meat, too few vegetables and fibre, too much processed food and too much sugar (without even knowing it – they put it in everything these days, including tomato sauce). I also wasn't drinking enough water. In my mind, meat should be classified as processed food, simply due to how the animals are reared. Did you know that 80% of all antibiotics sold are used for animals?

My spaghetti bolognaise on Mondays was OK to a point. I added vegetables in the bolognaise sauce, but nowhere near the quantity to ensure I was getting the fibre I needed. The spaghetti was white, which meant that it didn't have enough fibre either, but tonnes of carbohydrates. I was cooking from scratch, but I was also using partially cooked tomatoes with herbs from a jar, so needless to say they contained added sugar and preservatives. As for the mincemeat, goodness only knows what drugs that cow had been injected with to mess with its hormones before it ended up on my plate to proceed to mess with mine. The same thing went for the chilli con carne. The only difference was that I was having white rice rather than spaghetti, with most of the goodness sucked out of it. So again there wasn't enough fibre. The pork chops were fine apart from I'd had red meat three days in a row and ingested whatever drugs the pig had consumed. The grilled fish was fine, but it was farmed, so no doubt it had been fed lots of interesting stuff that I didn't want to know about.

My objective is not to make you paranoid about food, but to try and inform some of your choices and help you make simple changes. On my healing journey, I decided to do the following:

» **Throw out everything white**

Bread, pasta, rice, tortilla wraps, etc. Switch to their brown equivalents. This helped me increase my fibre intake. I had such fun with rice, as there are so many varieties of it when you decide to move away from white. I love to mix the different colours together. For example, red, black and red. Just looking at the mixture of colours makes me want to eat it. I know people find cooking brown rice a challenge, but in my view if you can cook white rice, you can cook brown rice, it's just a matter of doubling the cooking time from 20 to 40 minutes. My health is definitely worth the additional time.

» **Go sugar free whenever possible**

No one can be 100% sugar free because it's present in fruit and honey, etc., but if you have to have sugar, have it in as natural a state as possible. That way you'll get the other nutrients as well. I went completely sugar free for one year and it was eye opening. Carrots had never tasted so good. This is because my taste buds were reset so everything tasted sweeter. The warning here is that before long you will not be able to eat your normal shop-bought cakes because they will taste too sweet.

Eat whole foods * Eat whole foods * Eat whole foods

They still have all the goodness. If you take nothing away from this book but to switch your diet to whole foods, you will be winning.

» **Eat organic wherever possible**

I know it is more expensive, but so are the healthcare bills and the drugs that are killing you.

» **Eat three proper meals a day**

This means making time for breakfast. Do not skip it. It will mess with your blood sugar levels and make you crave rubbish food. If you are eating the right foods, you will be fuller for longer and you won't need to snack between meals.

» Half your plate should be vegetables

Always ensure half your plate is just vegetables, especially the green leafy ones. This is huge! It will help you control your carbohydrate intake, which in turn affects weight gain. I used to be a real carb head and I was convinced I'd starve unless half my plate was filled with them. Then I started doing the half vegetables thing, which meant there wasn't enough room on the plate for my carb load, as I had to make room for protein as well. To my surprise, I literally reduced my carb intake per meal by three quarters and not only didn't I die, I felt just as full. The vegetables were indeed filling. If you are a carb head, trust me on this – you will not die. Have wholemeal carbs instead and you will do just fine.

» Drink two litres of water a day

I really need to go to town on this water thing, so here goes.

Hydration

I was one of those people with a phobia of public toilets. Seriously! Before I had children, I would only use them on the pain of death. To get around my issue, I'd avoid drinking too much fluid. I'd normally have a glass of water with my meal and that was it. When water became fashionable, and every celebrity worth their salt was clutching bottled water as an accessory, this lady was not for turning. Why would I want to subject myself to peeing all the time? What was that about? I convinced myself the water thing was a fad and I wasn't ever going to buy into it. Did I mention earlier that I used to suffer from constipation? I was eating the wrong carbs with not enough fibre and I also wasn't drinking enough water. I don't know what I was thinking, but if anyone should have been guzzling down water it was me, but I was busy in denial. As far as I was concerned, there were people in Africa who lived despite not having access to drinking water all the time, and it was hot there too. I decided this whole water thing was a marketing gimmick by Evian and I wasn't going to fall for it. But my body knew better and wasn't letting me off lightly. I got cramps a lot in the middle of the night and had tried all sorts to ease it, including rubbing magnesium gel into my thighs and scoffing bananas (not at the same time mind). To some degree or another, we all have a pill-popping mentality. We would rather pop a pill than change our lifestyle. Luckily for me, someone just mentioned in passing that cramps could be caused by dehydration. The irony was that we were in Houston, Texas, on a business trip during summer, when the temperature was off the charts. For some reason, I paid attention and that was goodbye to cramps and constipation.

Below are the benefits of drinking water. It:

- Keeps the body's fluids in balance. These are needed for essential functions, including: digestion, absorption, circulation, saliva creation, the transportation of nutrients and the maintenance of body temperature.

- Helps to control calories, as water is consumed instead of other sugary drinks.

- Energises muscles by maintaining the balance of fluid and preventing muscle fatigue.

- Keeps the skin looking good and prevents dehydration, which makes the skin look dry and wrinkled.

- Helps to support normal kidney function and cleanses and rids your body of toxins.

- Helps to maintain normal bowel function. When you don't get enough fluids, your colon pulls water from your stools in order to maintain hydration, and this results in constipation.

The jury is still out on how much water we should drink. It was previously thought that it should be two litres, but that figure doesn't seem to have any scientific basis. As a rule of thumb, your urine should flow freely, be light coloured and odour free. If you can work out the water intake quantity that helps you achieve all of the above, then good for you. The rest of us mere mortals can stick to the two litres until we do our own personal measurement. The bottom line is to keep hydrated and give your body a chance to function optimally and get rid of toxins.

Thankfully, I got my head out of my derriere about the water issue and I haven't looked back since. Here is how I get my intake. I am a very organised person, and I like my routines and lists. I worked out a way to incorporate the two litres into my day without getting caught short on the motorway. I had to get over my phobia of public toilets somewhat, but I am still not out of the woods. At work, I always have to use the same cubicle and still draw the line at real public toilets, such as the ones found in shopping centres. I know I need therapy, but I am busy working on my 14 other symptoms for now, so the phobia can wait in the queue. Anyway, this is what I do to stay hydrated. I find drinking plain water very boring and hot water is better for your digestion, so I drink tea instead. There is also the small win of not succumbing to bottled water. People have enjoyed tea for generations…it hasn't just become popular because the latest stick thin model has been seen clutching it. (After all, there are ceremonies around drinking tea.) That said, not any old tea will do, as you don't want to overload on caffeine either. I normally choose herbal tea. I put a couple of bags in my thermos travel mug and add hot water at drinking temperature. The thermos more or less keeps it at the same temperature and then I simply top it up with more hot water throughout the day. It is very easy to hit two litres that way. I can practically hit a litre and a half before noon. I believe my cup takes about 475ml, so I have one first thing after waking up. It is good to have a hot drink first thing in the morning, as it wakes up your digestive system. I sometimes mix it up and have hot water and lemon rather than herbal tea. Thirty minutes after breakfast, I start sipping my next batch. Then at around 10:30am to 11am, I start on the next one, with the aim of finishing before lunchtime. I start sipping again about 30 minutes after lunch, and get two more batches in that way, starting on the final one 30 minutes after dinner. See, if I'm being good, I can easily exceed the two-litre mark. I also have fun with the teas and try all sorts of weird herbal ones, so long as they don't contain caffeine. I hope this will encourage you to start drinking more water. By the way, I stop drinking about 30 minutes before eating and start drinking 30 minutes after eating, to avoid diluting my digestive fluids.

Accidental Weight Loss

As part of my health journey, I started eating breakfast, which after years of having this important meal on the go, was a real chore. Additionally, because I was now ensuring half my plate was made up of vegetables, by the time I had done my carbs, protein and good fats, my portion sizes were bigger than normal and yet I went down one belt hole without even trying.

It is interesting to note that I didn't change my way of eating in order to lose weight. To be honest, I have never had a weight problem (please don't hate me), so I was really surprised by my shrinking waistline, as I was eating a lot more than I did normally. My plate was now covered with a lot more vegetables and I was including all sorts of nuts and seeds in my salads, which I didn't do before.

Let me give you an example. Thursdays in the office is curry day. There are normally two different types of curry on offer, plus white rice, onion bhaji, naan bread, poppadoms and then some sort of condiment like mango chutney (packed full of sugar). Unfortunately, this is the office canteen so there is nothing I can do about the fact that the rice is white, so I live with that compromise. I normally go for the vegetarian curry, which will include two different types of bean curry. The rice fills up my carb allowance, so I don't touch the poppadoms and naan bread. Instead, I go to the salad bar and fill the other half of my plate with salad, including in it pumpkin and sunflower seeds. I also leave out the onion bhaji because although it started out as a vegetable, it has been fried and had all sorts added to it. As tasty as it is, I have no more room on my plate. This is how the weight loss happens. By default I am eating less carbs and less sugar, purely because I am switching them for salads. If someone had just told me to cut my carb consumption by half, it would have been hard to wrap my head around. But because my objective is to fill half my plate with vegetables, I automatically reduce my carb intake without feeling deprived.

I came to the low carb movement very late indeed…a bit like I did with the water thing. It's fair to say I am a bit of a late developer. I just saw it as yet another fad following the Atkins diet, and because I never had weight issues and didn't do diets, I just wasn't paying attention. Until, that is, I read Gary Taubes' book, *Why We Get Fat: And What To Do About It.* That was an eye opener! Again, this is not a book that would normally find its way onto my reading list. However, it was recommended to me because of its coverage on how carbohydrates affect our body. As I was on a health journey, I thought finding out more about this wasn't going to hurt. Well, if nothing, it explained why I lost the weight. The science in there about carbohydrates is very impressive stuff. In a nutshell, our insulin levels rise when we consume easily digestible carbohydrates and this prevents the body from burning fat for fuel. Foods such as refined carbohydrates in flour, cereal grains, potatoes and sugar drive us to amass fat.

There is a saying that 'when people know better, they do better'. This really applies to food. Once you know more about food and what your body needs, you make different choices. I began to have fun with my food. I got creative. Sometimes people look at my plate and wonder if we're eating from the same canteen. But it's simply about knowing more about food and how to put things together. You owe it to yourself to examine your diet, take out the things that don't serve you and pack it with all the good foods that will give you health. Interestingly, this approach works for everything in life, too, as you will see in the other chapters.

CHAPTER SEVEN

ARE YOU SLEEPING THROUGH LIFE?

Early to bed early to rise, makes a man healthy, wealthy and wise.

~ BENJAMIN FRANKLIN

Physical Part 2: Sleep and Exercise

Sleep

One in three people set more than five separate alarms in order to wake up on time in the morning. Despite this, the average snooze time clocks up to 14 minutes. To me, this is 14 minutes of torturing yourself because once your alarm goes off, you never really go back to sleep. You're in the land of being half asleep and half awake and neither state wins. Then there is the guilt that nags at you and says, 'you really should be awake'. Followed by the blame when you finally drag your sorry behind out of bed and then run into traffic.

For years I convinced myself I wasn't a morning person. I was one of those people who would rather stay up late watching crap TV and wake up with the TV watching me. Then I would stumble upstairs and then struggle for a lifetime to fall asleep again, only to wake up (what felt like) ten minutes later. When I discovered I had to aim for eight to nine hours' sleep every night, I was staggered. How does anyone ever get eight hours' sleep? If only we listened to our bodies. I was falling asleep in front of the TV because I was constantly exhausted and the moment I sat down, I went straight to the land of nod. Fatigue was one of my 14 symptoms. It is amazing how many of us live with this tiredness and accept it as the norm. A doctor once told me that I had small children and worked full-time so the fatigue was to be expected. Seriously? How about for starters just having enough sleep?

My chronic fatigue was down to my hormone imbalance, which made me oestrogen dominant. This led to fibroids, which led to heavy bleeding, which led to iron deficiency, which led to tiredness. By the way, I found all this out by myself. Yes, pat me on the back if you like, but it has been a hard-won fight. Now, guess what contributes to hormone imbalance? Lack of sleep! Basically, if you don't get enough hours in, you put your body under stress, and stress messes with your hormones. In the winter of your cycle, the first seven days are when you need to ensure you get as much rest as possible. This is not the time for late-night *Game of Thrones* binge-watching sessions. Working on your sleep is not like taking HRT, jacking up your hormones, becoming a horny old goat overnight and living with the drug's side effects. It is a change in lifestyle to deal with underlying health conditions and it can take a while to see the benefits. But when they do kick in, they are holistic, efficient and don't throw other parts of your health off-kilter. That said, fixing your sleep is the quickest way to increase your energy levels. For me, even though I had the additional issue of iron deficiency, once I got the sleep thing sorted, I stopped dropping off in front of the TV. I'd still get extremely tired in the second part of my luteal phase and be completely wiped out after my period, due to the amount of blood I had lost, but I was able to bounce back quicker. My chronic, unrelenting fatigue had made everything feel like an uphill battle.

The relationship between sleep and health

Over the page are some research findings from the Harvard University division of sleep medicine:

- **Obesity**

  During sleep, our bodies secrete hormones that help to control appetite, energy, metabolism and the processing of glucose. Lack of sleep increases the production of cortisol, the stress hormone.

  As an aside, remember there is an increase in cortisol in the second part of your luteal phase, the week before your period. Can you see how lack of sleep can lead to heightened PMT? Anyway, back to the obesity.

  For someone who is lactose intolerant, whenever I am stressed, ice cream suddenly becomes a must have. You don't need me to tell you that lack of sleep affects decision-making abilities. Anyway, back to the science. Lack of sleep increases the production of insulin, which promotes fat storage. So not only am I eating the ice cream, I am also storing it.

  It gets worse: lack of sleep also results in the production of lower levels of the hormone leptin, whose job it is to alert the brain that it has had enough food.

  More ice cream.

  Then, to add insult to injury, higher levels of the biochemical ghrelin is produced. Ghrelin stimulates appetite. It may also make you more likely to reach for foods that will satisfy your craving for a quick energy boost, such as sweets.

  So, even more ice cream. All because you didn't have enough sleep.

  Then, in my case, after all that ice cream, I end up with stomach ache and bloating and go on to look three months pregnant for the next 24 hours because of the lactose intolerance. Ideal!

- **Diabetes**

  Lack of sleep adversely affects the way the body processes

glucose, the high-energy carbohydrate that our cells use for fuel, and this can lead to type 2 diabetes.

- **Heart disease and hypertension**

There is a correlation between lack of sleep and cardiovascular disease and stroke. Research found that people with hypertension who had a single night of poor sleep experienced elevated blood pressure levels throughout the following day. Chronic elevation of blood pressure can lead to cardiovascular disease.

- **Mood disorders**

Chronic sleep issues have been linked with depression, anxiety and mental distress. In one study, subjects who slept for four hours per night showed declining levels of optimism. By the way, all these symptoms improved when the subjects returned to a normal sleep schedule.

This is the easiest one to test without science. We all know that if we don't have enough sleep, we feel tired and irritable the next day.

- **Immune function**

We naturally want to sleep when we're unwell. It turns out that substances produced by our immune system when fighting infection induce fatigue. It is as if your immune system needs you to be asleep so that it can do its thing. Studies in animals have also verified that people who get some deep sleep following an infection have a better chance of survival.

- **Alcohol**

Lack of sleep can make you more prone to turn to alcohol. One reason for this is that people with sleep problems might reach for booze because of its sedative properties. The other reason is that alcohol-induced sedation is only temporary and as the effects wear off, you will wake up again, which can lead to other sleep problems.

- **Life expectancy**

  Considering all the above, it's no surprise that lack of sleep has an adverse effect on life expectancy. Data from three large studies suggest that sleeping five hours or less per night increases our mortality risk from all causes by roughly 15%.

Hopefully, the above has now convinced you to take your sleep seriously. Below are some tips to help you along your good sleep journey:

1. **Avoid caffeine, alcohol, nicotine and other chemicals that interfere with sleep for four to six hours before you go to bed.**

   I can't be bothered to count the hours, so I just avoid caffeine.

2. **Turn your bedroom into a sleep-inducing environment.**

   No flickering lights, no TV, blackout blinds, no phones…you get the drift.

3. **Establish a pre-sleep routine.**

   You can really go to town on this, especially in the winter part of your cycle – the first seven days – when you are supposed to be in full-on self-care mode. Have a bath, light some scented candles, read a book or listen to soothing music. This is your chill-out time. Sometimes you may need to fight for it, but remember that you are worth it.

   Avoid strenuous exercise or stressful emotional conversations. I used to bottle up everything that upset me during the day and then offload onto my husband at bedtime. He said I always used to come to bed angry. I can't think why, but now I know better and I protect the sanctuary of my bedroom and try hard to leave my crap at the door. Before I adopted this habit, interestingly enough, I would not allow a TV in the bedroom, but I would go in there and yell before bedtime because a child had left a sock on the stairs!

4. **Go to bed when you are tired rather than allowing yourself to fall asleep on the sofa.**

If you go to bed and have not fallen asleep within 20 minutes, get up and engage in a quiet, restful activity. Reading is a good one.

My suggestion is to meditate (more on this later). There is nothing that will put you to sleep faster, as most of us suddenly feel like sleeping the moment we have to meditate. In fact, I got into meditation originally when my father died and I experienced sleep terrors. The objective was to calm my mind down so that I could sleep without it ticking over and tipping me into experiencing terror.

5. **Keep your watch/clock out of sight.**

Watching the clock tick is not going to make you fall asleep. It'll stress you out and you'll be in trouble once you get the cortisol going. Ensure your watch/clock isn't visible. If you use your phone like me, ensure it's not flashing at you and you can't see the time. You should always put it on silent so only the alarm will ring.

6. **Use natural light to your advantage because it will help to set your body clock.**

Let in the light in the morning. I am one for opening windows and curtains. If there is natural light out there, I am having it. I don't care what sophisticated lighting a building has – I will squeeze the last drop out of any natural light.

Go out in the afternoon when the sun is out. Apart from the effect on your body clock, you'll also top up on Vitamin D, which is an added bonus.

7. **Keep your internal clock set with a consistent sleep schedule.**

   This is huge! If you don't do any of the above, do this one. This is the one I stuck to as if my life depended on it, and it paid off.

   You are aiming for the optimum eight-nine hours' sleep every night, so set your sleep window and stick to it. I do the 10pm-6am. I have tried different windows. 11pm-7am or 9pm-5am, but they didn't work as well for me. Find out what works for you and stick to it. It will soon become automatic and you will start beating your alarm clock.

8. **If you must take a nap, nap early.**

   Some people find that they get tired during the day and need a nap. If you must nap, make sure it is over by 5pm; any later than that and your sleep will be disrupted.

9. **Make your evening meals light and ensure your last meal is three hours before you go to sleep.**

10. **Watch your fluid intake.**

    You want to drink enough to stay hydrated, but not too much, which will disrupt your slumber. I stop drinking 30 minutes before I go to sleep.

11. **Try to finish exercise three hours before bedtime. Working out produces cortisol, which keeps you alert and you don't want that before bedtime.**

    I prefer to exercise first thing in the morning, just to get it out of the way so I can get on with my day. I exercise because I have to, not because I am a fitness fanatic. To be honest, I do the minimum I can get away with, which is 30 minutes a day. I know myself and I'll try and find any excuse not to work out, so tackling it first thing works out best for me. My husband, meanwhile, prefers to exercise at lunchtime. You have to find the time that works for you and make sure it is three hours before your bedtime.

For me, the results of having more sleep were revolutionary. I must say, I was quite disciplined about this and was in bed by 10pm most nights, with my alarm set for 6am. I've never had a problem with dropping off to sleep (I tell my husband it is the result of having a clean conscience), but my problem used to be waking up in the morning. I don't have that problem anymore. I promise you, it had nothing to do with self-discipline. You can be self-disciplined all you want, but if your body is not getting enough rest then you are setting yourself up for more frustration. You need to be well rested before you can wake up feeling that you can take on the world and be the superwoman that you are.

When I got my sleep sorted, a surprising thing started to happen.

Every morning before this, my alarm clock would yank me out of my deep sleep, almost giving me a heart attack. Following this, I would leap up and slam the off button on the head. I would then go back to that sort of half sleep, where you are not really asleep but you don't want to wake up either because you are pissed off with your alarm and everything else, even before the day has started. These days, though, I wake up naturally maybe 10 minutes before the alarm clock goes off and just lay there listening to the birds chirruping away (or battling my thoughts, but more on that later). When my alarm goes off, there is no shock or leaping involved, as I've been expecting it. This means I don't wake up pissed off first thing, my day has a chance of being pretty decent and I'm more likely to be objective in situations, rather than behaving like I got out of the bed on the wrong side.

I can't tell you what a huge difference this has made to my life. I wake up feeling more rested, less hurried and more in control. Just try it for yourself. Set yourself a bedtime that allows you to have 8 hours' sleep and stick to it. Then just watch the change in your energy levels and your mood.

We have discussed what you should eat and drink and when you should sleep, now let's get onto exercise.

Exercise

Those who think they haven't got time for bodily exercise
will sooner or later have to find time for illness.

- EDWARD STANLEY

Let me let you into a little secret. I hate exercise. There, I've said it! In fact, given half a chance, I would not do anything that involved sweating. I was lucky to get away with my lack of exercise for as long as I did. Even now it doesn't come naturally to me. I had good eating habits to a point and thanks to my lactose intolerance and not having a sweet tooth, I somehow managed to get away with very little exercise until I started having my health problems. I guess my redeeming quality is that I have always loved to walk. I could walk until my legs fell off, and my dogs can attest to that. I also love yoga and there is a set of yoga exercises I do most mornings, but that is hardly breaking into a sweat. My yoga exercises are not the high-octane, Ashtanga type ones that were all the rage a few years ago. Mine are the namby-pamby type, which are meant to energise and balance the energies in my body, enabling me to sit still for meditation. So no, balancing-my-whole-body-weight-on-a-fingernail-while-touching-my-third-eye is not my type of yoga, if you get my drift. Gyms are still a bit of a mystery to me. I will think nothing of wearing half my wardrobe to walk my dogs through rain, sleet and snow and coming back covered in mud. On the other hand, I balk at wearing Lycra and leaping about while others pretend not to notice my flailing limbs in a gym. You get the point. I am, however, what I would call a functional exerciser. When I worked in Central London, to ensure I got a daily walk into my routine, I would get off at the station before my stop and walk for 30 minutes to the office. I used to get in an hour's exercise, as I would do this after work too. As you get older, though, you need to add in a bit of resistance training, which is good for your bones. I speed walk now just so that I can get the sweat in, and I keep threatening to get my husband to show me how to do some weights, as he does them avidly. I aim to do at least 30 minutes of exercise a day. The rule is this has to involve a little sweat – not too much, mind. I got over my sweat issue when I learnt that you get rid of toxins by sweating. Give me the health reason for why I should do something I don't like and suddenly I don't mind doing it so much.

Find the time that you are most likely to exercise and do it. I know that if I don't exercise in the morning, it will never happen. I also like the way it makes me feel. Afterwards, I feel like I can take on any challenge. It sets me up. I am not one of those people who can come home from work, get their gym stuff on and head out. I tried exercising at lunchtime like my hubby, but I prefer to chat to my mates and the gym got in the way of this. The point is, know your optimum exercise window and utilise it. It doesn't matter what you do, just do something to start with, and, as time goes on, you will get fancy and start getting sweaty and thinking about weights. The most important thing is to build an exercise habit. If you know you'll be exercising at 7am every morning, for example, the content will take care of itself. Luckily for me, my dogs will not let me off. They follow me around in the morning until I take them out.

Benefits of exercise

If you need more reasons to exercise, here are some figures from the NHS website. It's medically proven that people who do regular physical activity have up to:

- A 35% lower risk of coronary heart disease and stroke

- A 50% lower risk of type 2 diabetes

- A 50% lower risk of colon cancer

- A 20% lower risk of breast cancer

- A 30% lower risk of early death

- A 83% lower risk of osteoarthritis

- A 68% lower risk of hip fracture

- A 30% lower risk of falls (among older adults)

- A 30% lower risk of depression

- A 30% lower risk of dementia

Unfortunately, exercise is not a pill that we can just swallow and reap the benefits from, but if a pharmaceutical company came up with a drug that did all of the above, it would be the most cost-efficient pill ever invented. Additionally, it wouldn't have any adverse side effects.

What a bonus!

Let's delve into the benefits of exercise that are most beneficial for women.

1. **Reduces your risk of dementia by 30%**

   According to a report by Public Health England (PHE), Alzheimer's disease and dementia are the biggest causes of death among women.

   Staying active boosts cognitive function and energy levels, thereby reducing the risk of developing dementia. I have just lost my mother-in law who suffered from dementia for a few years before she died. It was heartbreaking to watch a vibrant, intelligent woman succumb to such a cruel illness. She had so much to give and was robbed of all that in her final years.

2. **Decreases the risk of osteoporosis**

   Osteoporosis is a disease in which bones become fragile and more likely to break. It is most prevalent in post-menopausal women.

   Remember the hip pain I had from Great Portland Street tube station? According to my Harley Street consultant, my bone density left a lot to be desired. Did I also mention that I could take or leave exercise at that time of my life because I didn't do sweat?

   Strengthening exercises such as weightlifting, jogging, hiking, stair climbing, step aerobics and dancing-related sports are the best. I cannot wait until I get an opening in my life so that I can take up ballroom dancing. I am normally glued to the TV in the winter when *Strictly Come Dancing* comes on. Suffice to say, I love dancing and I am the first one up on the dance floor at any social function, embarrassing as that may be for my kids. Dancing is good for the bones, but it's also good for the soul. Next time you are out and there is the opportunity to dance, just get on there and do it for your bone density. Go ahead and shake what your mama gave you. You know it makes sense.

3. Improves sex life

Research from the Harvard School of Public Health found that just 20 minutes of regular exercise a day can improve sexual response in women. Yale's University Prevention Research Center echoes the same point.

Ladies, need I say more? We all know how much our peace of mind is hinged on a good sex life. Not least because without it, another person can easily come into the relationship, or the partnership may dissolve altogether. Sex simply oils the wheels of a relationship. Don't get me wrong, I for one think that if a woman is not putting out, the partner has a responsibility to grin and bear it until Her Royal Highness is in the mood. That said, some of us, left to our own devices, what with hormone imbalance issues and chronic fatigue, would never be in the mood. That is a recipe for friction and resentment from the other party, even though they have agreed 'till death do us part'. I don't think holding out on sex is remotely near the realm of death, but it might not feel like that to our partners. Unfortunately, implicit in the 'till death do us part', silent though it might be, is also the 'to have sex till death do us part'. So hormonal imbalances notwithstanding, for peace of mind, it behoves you to get the exercise going just so that at the very minimum you can fulfil your marital duties. Hopefully once said duties have been met you can then focus on the enjoyment sex.

4. Prevents muscle loss

If you want to look good and toned in your summer dress, then you have to build muscle. Exercise helps to increase muscle mass and contributes to healthy aging. If your legs are flabby you won't exactly be able to pull off the Angelina Jolie leg stance in that evening gown with the slit to the thigh.

5. **Improves digestion**

   Exercise helps the intestinal muscles break down food and move it through the digestive tract correctly by strengthening the abdominal muscles and minimising sluggishness. If your digestive system is suboptimal, this will impact the way you absorb nutrients from your food. So you can be eating your rather expensive organic, grass fed beef, or corn fed chicken, and swallowing enough vitamins to block your kitchen drain, but still not benefiting from the full benefits of your healthy diet.

   I hate exercise. Have I said that already? Well, indulge me again. I am prone to digestive issues and constipation, so for me failing to exercise is no longer an option. I may not be in the gym leaping from one piece of equipment to the other, but I will at least go for a brisk walk. Anyone can fit a 30-minute fast walk into their day.

6. **Reduces stress, depression and anxiety by 30%**

   This is particularly important for women, who demonstrate an incidence of depression that is reported to be almost double that of men in both developed and developing countries. I gave these figures in my opening chapter. Depression is the second most common cause of ill health among women.

   Neurotransmitters and endorphins that ease depression are released during exercise. Additionally, the body temperature becomes raised, which has been shown to calm nerves.

   Next time you experience any emotional turbulence, aka PMS, when you are in the autumn of your cycle in the week preceding your period, try some digging in the garden (if you have one), it'll beat stabbing your loved ones in the eye and it will work wonders for your mood. If not, you can always go for a brisk walk or a run around the park.

Someone told me once that you never see a depressed person walking fast. It stands to reason that if you are depressed, you will not be full of the joys of spring and bouncing off the pavements. So maybe we shouldn't allow ourselves to get that far down. We need to build an exercise habit into our routine in order to release all those happy endorphins, whether we need them or not.

7. **Reduces breast cancer risk by 20%**

According to the World Health Organisation (WHO), breast cancer is the mostly commonly diagnosed cancer in women.

In fact, a 2007 study found that exercise is an important step to preventing breast cancer because higher levels of oestrogen (which is stored in fat) increase your risk. It is a well-known fact that sports women tend to have irregular periods due to all the exercise they do. I am not advocating irregular periods, as this comes with its own problems, but normal women just need their normal dose of oestrogen in order to have a normal monthly cycle.

I was oestrogen dominant for years. To add insult to injury, I avoided exercise because I simply didn't know any better. (I didn't have a weight issue so I didn't see the point.) Looking back now, it's hard to believe that I once thought like that. If you now add to the mix the fact that I had digestive issues, wasn't drinking enough water or eating enough fibre, my body's elimination process was not the best to get rid of the excess oestrogen. Was I not the perfect candidate for hormone imbalance issues?

By the way, the risk of both lung and colon cancer are also increased by lack of exercise.

8. **Reduces the risk of coronary heart disease and stroke by 35%**

   According to the World Health Organisation (WHO), cardiovascular diseases account for one-third of deaths among women around the world, and half of all deaths in women over 50 in developing countries. This is a staggering figure. Basically, 30% of deaths in women living in developed countries could be slashed to 20% if we put our trainers on and headed out for some exercise.

9. **Improves your skin**

   There is nothing more ageing than wrinkles. Exercise enhances the blood flow to your skin and lends it a youthful look. It also improves bad skin by controlling the production of acne-inducing testosterone hormones, such as DHEA and DHT. Additionally, sweating helps you get rid of toxins and clears your pores.

   I don't know about you, but I certainly want youthful and glowing skin. Couple this with optimal hydration and you will be positively glowing.

CHAPTER EIGHT

THE WORLD YOU LIVE IN

Our environment, the world in which we live and work,
is a mirror of our attitudes and expectations.

~ EARL NIGHTINGALE

Physical Part 3: Environment

For now the focus is on our physical environment. We will get into the mental later. When it comes to environment, my motto is: simplify, simplify, simplify. Cut out the clutter. If you haven't used it in a year, chances are that you will never use it, so get rid of it. Isn't it about time you freed yourself from that dated fondue set you have been stumbling over for years? You need to make room for a Kombucha (fermented tea) making set, which is now all the rage. Unless you want to keep moving house, you need to learn how to de-clutter and get rid of what doesn't serve you anymore. Incidentally, the week before your period is ideal for clearing your clutter. It works physically to combat the increase in cortisol that is making you feel a bit stressed. It'll give you a bit of exercise and provide a form of release, too.

In her book *The Happiness Project*, American author Gretchen Rubin goes through how she did her de-cluttering and how it impacted her life. The fact is that if you clear the clutter, AKA rubbish, from your environment, it will make room for you to see what you really have, and clear the way for fresher new things and a brighter perspective. I have a ritual where at the end of every year, I go through my wardrobe and the kids' wardrobes to clear out clothes for charity. I do this thinning out because I don't want to take rubbish into the new year.

I remember someone coming to my house once and asking: 'How do you keep everything so tidy and keep on top of it all?' The funny thing is that when I only had one baby, I went to someone's house and asked the same question. Anyone who knew me when I was growing up will tell you that I was the messiest kid alive. It was no better when I moved into my first flat. I always wanted a clean and tidy house but wasn't sure I wanted to do housework for all my waking hours. The key again is habit. Build habits that support your lifestyle; a bit like the exercise habit. If you build the habit of cleaning up after yourself, then cleaning up after dinner just becomes part of the habit. This also means you don't wake up to a dirty kitchen, with pots and pans everywhere. You may think that leaving a messy kitchen overnight doesn't matter, but it does – especially in the second half of your luteal phase. It will upset your sense of calm and wellbeing on some level. You won't feel it when you are at your most robust, but in the third week of your cycle, when you're at your most inward facing, you'll feel things more intensely. Clutter is mentally draining, but a lot of us have lived with that disturbance for such a long time we don't notice it anymore. That doesn't mean it has gone away. On some level it's still sucking up your energy. When you start living a balanced life, your tolerance for such disturbances will be lessened.

In a UCLA-published study called 'Life at Home in the Twenty-First Century', researchers observed 32 middle-class Los Angeles families and found that all of the mothers' stress hormones spiked during the time they spent dealing with their belongings. 75% of the families in the study had run out of space in their garages to park their car.

Another study at Yale School of Medicine found that two areas of the brain – the anterior cingulate cortex and the insula – are activated when hoarders have to let go of their stuff. This is the same area that is activated when smokers or drug addicts are trying to quit. This area is for pain and conflict and it's a very powerful neural signature.

Clutter is spiking your stress hormones and making you behave like an addict. This is not an efficient way to manage your life. Living well is about not allowing environmental factors to drain you of energy.

We all accept it is much nicer to relax in a tidy room than it is in a cluttered one. No one needs to read a book about that or trawl through statistics to be convinced. The more evolved you are as a person, the more you automatically move away from chaos in any form. Clutter is physical chaos.

As a woman, a working woman and a mother to boot, you don't have the luxury of 10 minutes in the morning to spend searching for a pair of socks. For you to fit in the lifetime of things you have to do before you go off to tackle the onslaught at work, you can't have a detour to look for something. Do yourself a favour and create a tidiness habit. Get the kids into that habit, too. If everyone cleans and tidies up after themselves, there will be less housework for you to do. Plus, you will be able to find things when you most need them.

Lots of offices now operate a clean desk policy. The corporate world cottoned onto the fact that people are more productive when they are not buried under clutter.

There are creatives out there who will swear blind that they need all their clutter to get their creative juices flowing. It doesn't matter what your style is so long as you are not activating any pain and conflict parts in your brain. Everyone has got a different clutter profile. This is similar to how some people like to live in Spartan environments while others enjoy the cottagey-things-thrown-together style. I have got no quarrel with that, but most of us are mere mortals and for us a clear desk means a clear mind.

I have given you the science about this, but putting science aside:

how do you feel when you walk into a messy room? How do you feel when you walk into a tidy room? How do you feel after you have gone to the trouble of tidying up a room? See, no science needed! Your energy levels should answer the question.

To get rid of clutter, you just need to create good tidying-up habits in order to keep on top of things. Here are some simple tips:

- Clear out the clutter periodically, e.g. once a year.

- Find a home for everything and keep everything in its home.

- Tidy up as you go along.

- Simplify wherever possible.

- If it's not of use, beautiful or of sentimental value, throw it out.

There are strategies and books written about this topic, and if you have a garage full of stuff you've accumulated over the years, you could find yourself clearing it out forever. Start small. Begin with a shelf in a cupboard, and see how good you feel when you've reorganised it. Then feed off the energy you've gained from doing that.

Your living environment, especially your home, is very important to your wellbeing, so give it the credit it deserves and you will find that you have a sanctuary in which to escape from the world.

So now that you are eating well, sleeping well, exercising and have turned your home into a sanctuary, what next? So far, these have all been physical, and although this is important, what goes on inside is even more important. Remember at the start of this book how I said I wanted to do things back to front on Maslow's pyramid, working from the spiritual downwards, but I didn't because I was afraid of losing people? To me, if the spiritual is right, the emotional and physical will be right too. Your philosophy on life affects how you interact with your environment and the people in it. If your house is cluttered, your mind is cluttered. If your mind is cluttered, you cannot see the wood for the trees. On the other hand, if you have formed the habit of right thinking and only allow thoughts that support you into your life, then this will lead you to clearing the clutter that is not serving you out of your kitchen or garage too. These things seem physical but you will soon find out that they are indeed psychological and if they are psychological, then they are spiritual.

So, onwards and upwards to the emotional.

CHAPTER NINE

PEACE OF MIND

When wealth is lost, you have lost a little, when health is lost, you have lost something of more consequence; but when peace of mind is lost, you have lost your highest treasure.

~ PARAMAHANSA YOGANANDA

Emotional: Part 1

Shall we start with some maths?

Peace of mind = emotional health.

We live in a wealth creation society. Somewhere along the line, we all bought into the propaganda that the more you have, the better you'll feel. We structured our lives accordingly and now we are paying the price with antidepressants. We have got the things all right, but we are still not happy. Also, the clutter those things created is now spiking our stress levels.

A landmark study by a team of researchers at the London School of Economics, which was based on data from Australia, Britain, Germany and the US, looked at responses from 200,000 people on how different factors impacted life satisfaction. Surprisingly, the big ones were non-economic! The table over the page shows the big hitters:

Position	Factors Impacting Life Satisfaction	% Of Measured Variance
1	Mental health (diagnosed depression/anxiety)	30%
2	Partnered	17%
3	Physical health (No. of conditions)	16%
4	Income	14%
5	Not employed	10%
6	Non-criminality	10%
7	Education	3%
		100%

Table 2. Life Satisfaction Table

Mental health, which controls our emotional state, is at the top and has an impact more than twice that of income. Physical health and being in a relationship are neck and neck, but again, both of them punch above income. So why do we sacrifice our relationships and our health to chase our career?

The findings don't stop there. They also found that the best predictor of an adult's life satisfaction is their emotional health as a child. You could be forgiven for glossing over this fact, but it gets better.

The same study published the different factors that affect a child's emotional health. On the next page is the ranking of the top four factors:

Position	Factors Impacting Outcomes	Emotional Outcome
1	Mother's mental health	54%
2	Family income	20%
3	Parent's involvement	14%
4	Father's mental health	12%

Table 3. Emotional Development

Isn't it eye opening that the mother's mental health has five times more of an impact than the father's? The effect of income is less than half that of the mother's mental health. Again, this is not to put women under pressure, but to highlight how pivotal we are to the future generation.

In chapter one, I gave you figures for how one in four women in the US and one in three in the UK take some sort of mental health medication. I also explained how depression and anxiety in women is twice as high compared to men. Yet it is the mental health of women that most affects the emotional stability of their children, and this is what impacts their happiness the most.

If you are stressed out and tired, the time you spend with your child is going to be fraught with tension, because you are operating from an emotional deficit. If this is your modus operandi, and your child is subjected to this day in, day out, then before you know it he or she will be on a psychologist's couch some 20 years later blaming you for all the ills of the world. I am not trying to pile on the pressure here. God knows, we women do that very well without any outside help.

The point I am trying to drive home here is that as women, we literally hold the happiness of the next generation in our hands, so we cannot afford to neglect ourselves emotionally. As the research also showed, we impact the wellbeing of our partners more than their income. Are you beginning to realise how instrumental your emotional health is on the world as a whole? At the risk of sounding political, it beggars belief that women and our emotional wellbeing are not at the centre of all political agendas. The phrase 'happy wife, happy life' has never been more true.

From research, we know the primary contributors to our wellbeing in order of highest contribution are:

- Mental Health
- Personal Relationships
- Physical Health

It is therefore confounding that society insists on laying so much importance on how much a person earns. Income is important but comes in at a dismal fourth in the pecking order. Perhaps this is because the impact of money is the easiest to see, like the big house or car. What use is a fancy job when you have got terminal cancer? Whereas if you lose your fancy job, so long as you've still got your health you can always get other work.

If we want to maximise happiness, our lives should be structured around prioritising emotional and mental wellbeing and our personal relationships. We should put a premium on family and doing what makes us feel good, rather than chasing the big pay packet. The emotional cost of working a job you hate with people you don't like is quite high and takes a toll on your body. You end up using the high pay packet to pay for your wrong choices. Additionally, it's not always guaranteed that the health damage due to poor choices can always be repaired, so why inflict the damage in the first place? Emotional health underpins how you manage your life. Ignore it at your peril. You cannot do all the physical things and ignore what is going on in your head.

Women are complex, emotional beings. Unfortunately, these days we medicate most of that emotionality away because we don't know how to manage it. We ignore the phases of our cycle. Our emotional nature, which is supposed to be a signalling system, is ignored for the most part just to enable us to navigate the stresses of modern-day living. This is a tragedy. Hillary Clinton was pilloried once for being tearful during her first presidential campaign. If you are a woman and you want to be taken seriously, you dare not show any soft emotions. Come to think of it, you dare not have a menstrual cycle.

We are not living the life we were designed to live. Imagine the chaos that would ensue if a traffic light system was shut down in a busy city because it was using too much energy? When we don't manage our emotional state, our traffic light system gets out of whack and it wreaks havoc with our sense of wellbeing. This is what happens when we don't respect our menstrual cycles and take time out for self-care. What's alarming is that rather than honour our cycle and ensure that we are emotionally stable, we would rather reach for the tablets or a bottle, or whatever is the easiest fix. Before we know it, we are on medication for our moods without even understanding most of the side effects. The result is that the edge is taken off life and we live through a fog, feeling disconnected from our true selves and our lives.

The top three contributors to life satisfaction are:

1. Mental Health
2. Personal Relationships
3. Physical Health

I will delve more deeply into mental health, which affects our emotional wellbeing, in the next chapter, so let's focus on the next two here:

Physical Health

Your physical health affects your emotional status, which in turn impacts your overall sense of wellbeing. Make up your mind that you are going to manage the physical contributors that are within your control. This is the first step to emotional health. I am going to assume now that after reading the previous chapters, you know what to do to take care of the physical. If you are healthy, the chances are your hormones won't be out of whack. Take it from someone who has lived with a hormone imbalance for years – if you wake up and you are hormonal, nothing anyone can do will make a difference. Your day can seem pointless. You wake up pissed off and go to bed even more pissed off. You feel anxious all the time but don't even know why. Your pre-menstrual tension becomes pre, post and during. There is simply no let up. I know because I've been there. Don't let things get that far. Nip it in the bud and take care of the physical. Eat right, hydrate, sleep right, exercise, schedule around your menstrual cycle and you'll be halfway there.

If you are unwell it can be stressful for you and the people around you, and it's not conducive to emotional wellbeing. Also, if the body is compromised, you can't do all the things you need to do to keep it in optimum working order to fight off disease. For example, you can't exercise if you are not feeling well. You will also want to eat rubbish, so it becomes a vicious cycle. You become constantly mildly unwell (I lived like that for a few years). You justify it to yourself that you are only carrying 14, shall we say, lifestyle symptoms. It's not as if your leg is hanging off, so you soldier on. You reason that none of your symptoms are serious enough to take you out. This may be true, but your energy is sucked out by those symptoms, which leaves you with no bandwidth to enjoy life. Take care of your physical health and your emotions will work for you.

People/relationships

This is a tough one. There you are, minding your own business when someone who is not managing their physical health and therefore is out of whack and emotional decides to come and be a pain in your backside. What to do? If this is at work, you can't fly off the handle because it will be considered unprofessional. If you are a female of a certain age, you are branded hormonal. If it is family, you can fly off the handle, but apart from getting it off your chest, what exactly does it achieve apart from pissing off your nearest and dearest? There is always the option of emigrating to Australia, but we can't all move to Australia to avoid our relatives. Even if you did, guess what? They have people in Australia, too, plus creepy crawlies. You have to find a way of dealing with people and keeping yourself on an emotional even keel. You have to manage your emotions.

I like to think I am a simple person. Others beg to differ but that is their problem. I like simplicity, as it helps me to make sense of life and, let's face it, life is complex. All this preamble is to lead you to a simple rule that I use:

If you don't make me feel good, there is no room for you in my life.

This doesn't necessarily mean the onus is on the other party to make you feel good. Take babies, for example. They don't do anything. You are the one doing all the caring, but they can give you a sense of purpose and make you feel loved unconditionally, etc. They make you feel good most of the time.

The question you need to ask yourself about the people in your life is whether they are adding or taking away from it. Relationships contribute to your emotional wellbeing, so if a person is not a positive influence, what the hell are they still doing in your life?

Of course, there are work colleagues that bug you, but you have to work with them. You know the ones. They…

- Have to make their voices heard and put ideas on the table without any thought as to how they will be achieved.
- Make you roll your eyes and ask God to give you strength.
- Don't want to do any work but want to throw their weight around and get all the praise.
- Have got their heads so far up the boss's behind that breathing is optional for them.

The sad thing is that they are everywhere you go. You can change jobs but if you don't come up with strategies to deal with these types you will forever be handing in your resignation.

Throw in the fact that women don't tend to be chest beaters. We don't normally enter the room proclaiming our achievements. Even if we know what we are doing, we still want to be doubly sure before we speak up. Have you ever sat in a meeting when a man has come up with an idea that you told him you were thinking about, only to hear him pass it off as his own without even a sideways glance of acknowledgement in your direction? I bet you have.

Here you are, hiding your light under a bushel while a colleague winds you up. And Australia is out of the question. What are you going to do?

First of all, you need perspective. Is it really as bad as you think? If you have taken care of your physical health and you are not hormonal then you can confidently say you are not overreacting. Half the time we lose our chance to deal with issues the right way because we aren't sure whether it is the time of the month or not. Sure, we all go through this time, but there are stupid, annoying people at every point in the month. So how are you going to manage this issue?

I am going to assume that you are not hormonal or paranoid because you respect the phases in your cycle and you are not off balance. Your physical health is also in tip-top shape.

You have to find out:

- Have you got the skills and language to speak up for yourself?

- Have you got what it takes to stop overthinking and not allow people to violate your boundaries?

- Do you even know where your boundaries are?

I have read several books on communication and the one that worked for me was *Nonviolent Communication* by Marshall B. Rosenberg.

The book goes through the four component parts of non-violent communication:

- Observations

- Feelings

- Needs

- Requests

Basically, this covers what our observations are of a situation, how this makes us feel, how we need to recognise what need in us is creating this feeling and how we can ask the other person to meet our need.

Here is an example:

When you ignore my project and focus on others in the team, it makes me feel taken for granted. I need to feel valued so I would appreciate it if in the future you could give me the same attention that you give to the others on the team.

This really is a language for life, and it is a tool you need in your arsenal to face the world every day. It works for colleagues, managers, husbands and children.

The magic is, once you learn to communicate and have those difficult conversations, you'll find that you don't have to change jobs as often or move Down Under. Additionally, your relationships become better because they are based on respect and you don't allow people to take you for granted.

The respect is on both sides, mind you. People know not to bring their bullshit your way because you have respectively defined your boundaries. On the other hand, you show others respect by not taking them out because you are feeling out of control.

There will always be people out there who will be chancing it and getting on your nerves. Sometimes, it will be because they don't know any better. At other times it will be because your self-care is lagging behind. You haven't exercised in a week and you've got several nerves exposed just waiting for some idiot to get on them. Sometimes, just sometimes, they might just be a pillock.

If you have mastered your ninja nonviolent communication strategies, you will feel equipped to handle them. You will have the confidence to negotiate and let your feelings be known without any casualties, including yourself. This will make you feel in control and let you reclaim your power. The following things will happen:

- You'll stem the negative flow of energy. You are not going to spend the rest of the day stewing over the fact that you didn't stand up for yourself. That stewing is not energy efficient and it puts you in a negative place.

- You'll feel proud for standing up for yourself.

- If the conversation goes right and the other person gets a chance to explain why they behaved that way, you will have learned something new about that person that will make for a better relationship in the future.

- Last but not least, you will have got it off your chest in a constructive way. Don't underestimate the value of that. Even if nothing else is achieved, this on its own is worth it. You can't always count on the other person being reasonable, but so long as you know you handled it responsibly, there is an inherent pat on the back in there. Try it...you will find yourself smiling silently to yourself.

Then it doesn't matter whether you are dealing with a child, a colleague in the office, your mother-in-law, or your child's teacher. It is the same principle. Put it in perspective, communicate it effectively and look for a way forward.

There will times when you'll be too angry to do any of the above. Take it from someone who has a lot of fire in her belly. I have a pact with myself; if I am too angry to deal with someone without using angry swear words then I leave it alone for 24 hours to cool down.

Every woman worth her salt needs to develop these skills. It is a survival skill. It keeps stupid people at arm's length, and it helps you get rid of toxic emotions. If you don't have an outlet for these, they eventually come out in an uncontrolled manner, which can expose you to a lot of damage limitation afterwards. Damage limitation – aka, I didn't manage my emotions and even though I started out in the right, I now have to apologise. This is just simply boring.

It took me a long time to accept the responsibility of managing my emotions. I thought the way you felt was just the way you felt and if you were upset, you were upset. I didn't accept the part I had to play in it. Do you know the expression: 'Someone has got your goat?' I am not sure where the goat came from, but it means you have allowed someone to get under your skin. The point of responsibility comes in when you realise your point of power. Someone cannot get your goat, or get under your skin, unless you allow them to.

When you are feeling unstable because you are not well, it is hard to accept that point of power. This is because you are not at your most powerful. So taking care of yourself is of the utmost importance. This way you are always in your power.

Tackling a difficult conversation when you are having your period and aren't feeling at your strongest isn't a wise move. When you are physically fit and you are not being drained by physical factors, it is easier to see your point of power. That said, unless you accept the responsibility and the part that you play in your emotions, you will not allow yourself to manage them.

Understand that you are not at your most articulate when you are so angry that your breathing is out of whack and you are jumbling your words. Surely it is better to come across as calm and measured? They do this in films sometimes when they let children say the most explosive things because it makes it extra shocking. It is the same with us. If you deliver something serious and important in a calm manner, it gives it more gravitas.

However, no matter how serious or important something is to you, if it is delivered in an angry manner people will find it easier to discount what you are saying by just labelling you as an angry person, even if what you are stating is perfectly valid. Manage your emotions and take control of your life. Give yourself a chance by taking that step back. Make up your mind that your emotions are there to power you on to achieve what you want rather than coming across as a raving lunatic. Trust me, everything feels different after 24 hours.

Without realising it, we all manage our emotions to some extent. When someone you love does something you don't like, you don't always fly off the handle, especially at the beginning of a relationship. You find ways to explain it away. When your toddler throws that bowl of cereal in your face for the third time, you somehow find the strength to wipe it off calmly without screaming. When your child is sick and you have been awake half the night dealing with poo and puke, you somehow manage to get up in the morning and take care of them and then go to work, albeit a bit grumpy. On top of that you manage to deal with a different bunch of grown up kids in the office. You have got what it takes to manage your emotions. You do it subconsciously and now all you have to do is manage it to your advantage. That enables you to come off as the cool customer you really are.

Abraham Lincoln said: *'Most people are as happy as they make up their minds to be.'*

When you make up your mind to be happy, you accept the responsibility for how you feel. This leads me onto a quote by Marcus Aurelius, the last of the five good Roman emperors:

'The happiness of your life depends on the quality of your thoughts.'

Let me put this in laywoman's terms. You cannot be happy if you are thinking rubbish thoughts. Here we go with the responsibility again! Your mood depends on what you are thinking. What you are thinking depends on how you are feeling, or is it the other way round? Food for thought!

This quote helped me to focus my thoughts on good things. There are tomes written about positive thinking and we will get to that when we get to the spiritual. For now, it's suffice to say that if you are thinking rubbish thoughts, your focus is on rubbish.

I personally think there is a flaw in how we were designed as humans. We should have been made to emit a foul smell whenever we think stinky thoughts. If that happened we would be forced to focus on good-quality thoughts, as no one wants to go around stinking.

I have got a thing about good quality. I hate cheaply made, poor quality stuff. I had to do a lot of work on myself not to get bogged down by perfectionism. I now know that good quality does not mean perfect. And besides, perfection does not even exist. For me, not thinking good-quality thoughts is bad on lots of levels. For starters, thoughts are something that I control and they are free, so why would I choose bad-quality thoughts while at the same time claiming I am all about quality?

I know a lot of people, including me, struggle with saying affirmations, which is a way of forcing good-quality thoughts to prevail, but there is another way. At any time when you become aware of your thoughts, just check the quality of them. Are you thinking about something that makes you feel good or are you stewing over that emotion you didn't express and now you can't get past it? It's easier to think good-quality thoughts when you express your emotions. If you are in your 24-hour cooling off period while you are angry about something, you have to channel your thoughts into something else that makes you feel good in the meantime. This takes effort and commitment. You will make the effort when you understand that your emotional state affects your wellbeing more than your salary.

Successful people think good-quality thoughts about the things that they are successful at. Women in good marriages think good-quality thoughts about their husbands. Sure, there are negative bits to their relationships, but that is not where their focus is. If you think you are good at something it is because your predominant thought about that thing is positive. Some people have a sunny disposition. I am not one of them, but ask anyone who knows me and they will tell you that I come across as a happy, positive person. It is because I choose good-quality thoughts because I understand their importance. I have had to work at this.

Positive thinking gets bad press sometimes, but here is a scenario:

Someone has upset you. They didn't do something the way you wanted them to do it, even though you have explained to them several times how you want it to be done. If you are anything like me, your usual internal chatter will kick in with something like:

Why don't people ever do what I want them to do?

Why do I always attract these sorts of people who want to take advantage of my good nature?

Why do people ignore my express wishes?

There must be something wrong with me.

Needless to say, these thoughts are coming from past hurts. Now I have been triggered and this could go on all weekend. Which means my kids and husband are going to have a *lovely* Saturday and Sunday.

Dare I say the person I am stewing about was probably having a bad day. A close relative is unwell, so perhaps they were a bit distracted. But never mind all that, the reasons why the person is ignoring my express wishes are neither here nor there. There will always be someone who is having a bad day. Am I always going to allow them to destabilise me and ruin everyone's weekend? Am I going to recognise my point of power and take my control back? Rather than going over the same old bad script in my head that I have played over and over again, am I going to change the script?

There is a fantastic book I read years ago called *What to Say When you Talk to Yourself* by Shad Helmstetter. In it he deals with the scripts we play to ourselves, why we do it and how to break the pattern.

This is where the quality of your thoughts comes in. Once you catch yourself thinking bad-quality thoughts, you have to change the script. Some people advise turning all the negatives into something positive. Well, that doesn't work for me and I find it a bit disingenuous to go from:

Why do people always take advantage of my good nature?

To

My good nature always attracts the best people to me!

I find it easier just to stop thinking those bad-quality thoughts and focus on something real in my life that is positive. It doesn't mean I don't deal with the situation and pretend it is not happening. Far from it, I just refuse to spend my weekend stewing over it.

Bad thoughts attract other bad thoughts (more on this later), so before I find my weekend ruined, I need to short circuit this run of bad-quality thoughts and go and think of something that makes me feel good. Then, come Monday, I will use my communication skills to deal with said issue. Also, by Monday, I will have enforced my 24-hour rule, calmed down and eliminated swear words, so I won't come across as a raving lunatic. Don't you just love killing two birds with one stone?

Other Relationships

Let's talk about the relationships that you have a choice over, such as the ones with friends – the ones you can walk away from. Who are you surrounding yourself with? I will go as far as to modify Marcus Aurelius's quote to read:

> 'The happiness of your life depends on the quality of your relationships.'

There is a natural phenomenon called osmosis. This is:

'A process by which molecules of a solvent tend to pass through a semipermeable membrane from a less concentrated solution into a more concentrated one.'

I am not going to get scientific about this, but just to point out the movement of molecules passing from less concentrated to more concentrated is mirrored in many aspects of life as well. Take note, it is not from more concentrated to less concentrated!

My interpretation of this is that if you surround yourself with positive people, you will become more like them. You will have access to more good-quality behaviours and thoughts to focus on.

We know how important it is to think good thoughts, as it affects the quality of our life, and just like misery loves company, good thoughts also love company. Depending on the spiral you want to go on, you make the choice regarding what you want to focus on – the power is in your hands. It does take some effort to acquire the skill of moving your focus to the positive whenever you become aware of your thoughts, but it's a really worthwhile endeavour. This is where meditation comes in. It helps you develop the skill of putting your attention where you want it to be. More on this later.

CHAPTER TEN

WHAT WAS I THINKING?

Cogito ergo sum. (I think, therefore I am.)
~ RENÉ DESCARTES

Emotional: Part 2

I am going to provide you with tools to help you manage your emotional wellbeing. Emotional wellbeing doesn't happen by accident. You have to take responsibility for your emotions. If not managed properly, certain things can make you feel out of control. Below are some key tools to help you win back control:

- Thought control

- Journaling

- Gratitude

- Time management

- Boundaries

Thought Control

Most of us never make the effort to control our thoughts. A stream of them run constantly through our minds and sometimes we pay attention to them and sometimes they are just doing their own thing.

It is quite hilarious when you try to pay attention to your thoughts. There is a lot of rubbish going on up there half the time, but we just don't notice. Just try paying attention to your thoughts for a minute and see what sort of things you are dwelling on. You will be surprised. Once you realise what goes on in your mind, trying to control your thoughts will not sound too alien.

In *The Buddha's Brain* by Rick Hanson, PhD, with Richard Mendius, MD, the two clever clogs go into the neuroscience of what is happening in the brain. They use the term: 'The negative bias of memory.' What does this mean exactly? Here is what they say:

> *'Your brain preferentially scans for, registers, stores, recalls and reacts to unpleasant experience…it's like Velcro for negative experiences and Teflon for positives ones. Consequently, even when positive experiences outnumber negative ones, the pile of negative implicit memories naturally grows faster. Then the background feelings of what it feels like to be you can become undeservedly glum and pessimistic.'*

What do I say to all this cleverness? You need to focus on the positive because the negative takes care to propagate by itself. That is the way we are built and it is a survival mechanism. You can't afford to give your brain free rein, otherwise you will just allow it to continue with its negative bias, which means you will be held hostage by negative thoughts.

Make yourself a promise that whenever you become aware of your thoughts, you will drag them somewhere positive and focus on something nice…something that makes you smile. In my view, this is different to positive thinking. There are people who tyrannise themselves into positive thinking and this can be quite draining and unsustainable. They literally try and pretend that the bad stuff isn't happening. That is denial and not facing up to reality. Managing your thoughts is about your point of focus. By all means acknowledge whatever it is that is going on that you don't like, but then move your focus to your point of power. Move somewhere where you are the one in control and choosing what you want to focus on. You'll feel powerful just by giving a nod to whatever the negative is and saying to yourself, 'I see you but I am not going to allow you to hold me hostage.'

In Eastern philosophy, there is the tradition of chanting a mantra continuously whenever you get the chance. When I first came across this I thought it was insane. Why would someone want to repeat a mantra to themselves? Hadn't they got anything better to do? Well, here is why. Your brain, left to its own devices, will drag you down the negative alley and have you thinking crap. Most of us can't be bothered to think up positive stuff, so the path of least resistance is to take a positive mantra and repeat it to yourself whenever you get a chance. At the minimum, you are disrupting the brain from making more negative pathways. If you can take your thoughts somewhere that makes you smile, you will be doing even better.

Another reason why we want to control our thoughts is that thoughts attract other thoughts of the same frequency. It's a bit like birds of the same feather flocking together. All you need is for something bad to happen, then you'll start thinking of the time two and a half years ago when the same thing happened and why it always happens to you. Before you know it, you'll be on Prozac! OK, so I am exaggerating here, but you get where I am going with this. Take control of your thoughts before they take control of you.

Journaling

If you love writing, journaling is a great way of managing your emotions and thoughts. For starters, the process of writing something down helps you process it. It gives you the clarity that you don't get when things are just mulling around in your head.

It also serves the purpose of 'better out than in'. If you are going through your 24-hour curfew of cooling off and editing your swear words, you can write everything down, which will help you gain perspective. Writing is cathartic. It clears the way for you to move on.

These days, you don't even have to write something down, you can speak it onto an app. The premise is the same…better out than in. I prefer writing or typing, even though it is not always convenient. There is something about the physicality of writing or typing that helps with the processing of thoughts.

Gratitude

Lots and lots has been written about practising gratitude and people swear by changing their lives with their gratitude journals. I am more into a gratitude habit. I will later show you how your habits determine your life, but for now let's focus on forming a gratitude habit.

Sticking with the example of feeling upset because someone has not done something the way you asked them to do it, where exactly does the gratitude come in here? Well, we are into thinking good-quality thoughts, as we now know they affect the quality of our lives. If you are thinking good-quality thoughts then you are thinking about nice things. If you are thinking about nice things that happened in the past then it is easy to feel grateful for them, especially now the opposite is happening. Instead of being annoyed and stewing over whatever wasn't done well, can you think about when something was done well by somebody else or by the same person? Can you switch your focus to something that is going well and be grateful for that? When you do this, it instantly changes your energy patterns.

Positive thoughts are about things you are grateful for, and those thoughts will be high frequency and change your vibration from low to high. Once you move onto positive thoughts, they'll attract more thoughts on that same frequency and before you know it you'll be on a beach in the Bahamas. Now I know where I would rather spend my weekend – in my mind anyway!

It's almost perverse the way you can move from upset to gratitude and then to a beach in the Bahamas, but this is a habit that can be built through practice. The reward for this habit is a good quality of life simply because you are thinking good-quality thoughts. You are not just making a random list of things that you are grateful for at the end of your day, but you are making gratitude a way of life, which in turn affects the quality of your life. If there is a whiff of making lemonade out of lemons about this then that is exactly what it is. You cannot control everything in your life, especially how other people react to you, but you can control your own reaction. Are you going to put yourself back in control, change your focus, change the quality of what you are thinking and change your frequency? Then voila! Life is practically your oyster in a moment that could have triggered all sorts of unhealed hurts and had you feeling sub-optimal.

Changing the focus or the quality of your thoughts can be labour intensive at the start, but anything worth acquiring doesn't come easily. This is a new skill of moving your attention to good-quality thoughts rather than stinky ones. Allow your thoughts to serve you. Do not leave them to their negative bias. If you are not sure what a good quality thought is, then ask yourself:

'Does this make me feel good?'

If the answer is 'no' then choose a different thought. It really is that simple. The question is whether you will put in the effort to shift your thoughts when you have got yourself all worked up and triggered. I know in times like this, it definitely feels easier to keep stewing rather than put in the effort to switch your thoughts. Wallow at your own peril.

Choose what you want to focus on rather than allowing your mind to run amok. Your mind is like an errant child. Left to its own devices, you will go round and round in circles in a negative bias. (This ties into meditation, so more on this in Chapter 14.)

Time management

I once worked for a guy who used to carry on meetings as he was doing the school run. Some people call it multi-tasking, I call it madness. No one wins. The whole point of the school run is to have a laugh with the kids on the way to school. These days it is practically impossible to tear kids away from their screens to have a chat. The school run presents a good opportunity to ban the phone and just have a natter. In the days when I used to walk my kids to school, we used to take the long cut as opposed to the short cut so the journey lasted longer. This was their idea not mine. I used to wonder where my life was going in those few minutes while I waited for them to emerge from yet another shrub along the long cut while I tutted impatiently. Interestingly, though, those are the memories that the kids cherish. Imagine if I had been on the phone trying to be clever and hold a meeting at the same time. The emergence from a shrub would have been missed. Children always want to show their parents what they are doing. It may seem mundane to us, but the 'Hey, Mum, I am holding a twig' moment is laying emotional foundations, and saying 'I matter' to the child. It contributes to their self-esteem. They would have felt deprived of that emotional connection if I had been on the phone when they emerged out of the shrub, and the people on the phone would have also sensed they didn't have my full attention. How many of us will put our phone on silent in a business meeting, but when spending time with our kids anyone is allowed to interrupt? We should all be made to memorise the table in Chapter Nine regarding what impacts our happiness the most.

In our busy world, where we have got technology and can work on the run, we are more stressed out than ever. Rather than allocating time to a task, we try to shoehorn two tasks into the same slot, just because we can. That isn't clever; it's stressful and no one wins. The fact that we can doesn't mean that we should.

It is practically impossible these days to have a chat with someone for more than three minutes without some sort of interruption from a device. Undivided attention has become a rare commodity.

The tragedy of all this is that it is human connections that de-stress us. It is not the money we make. It is not the house. It is the sense of belonging. Social interactions contribute more to our wellbeing than doubling our income. So why are the social things the first to be compromised?

The very thing we are sacrificing because we are too busy is exactly what we need in order to de-stress.

Are we packing more into our day than we need to?

Are we multi-tasking when we should be focusing on one thing at a time and getting the full benefit?

Are we scheduling time in our day for the things that matter?

To live a successful life, we have to be aware of the things that are important to us and make us feel alive, then do more of those things.

If you take a cold, hard look at your week, you will be shocked by where you are expending your life energy. If you are constantly tired and drained and don't have enough energy for life, I can guarantee that you are spending more of your life energies on things that drain you and not on enough things that replenish you. I will also bet my bottom dollar that you are ignoring the phases of your cycle.

Some people are just bad planners and some people don't plan at all. They just stumble through life, do what they have to do and never take a stand to say: 'This is where I want to go.' If you are one of those people and it is working for you, I doubt you will have got this far with the book.

However, if you want to take control of your life and stop feeling like an octopus on a treadmill, arms flailing every which way with the ground underneath you shifting, then it is about time you thought seriously about how to manage your time. Structure your day, week, month and year in such a way that all elements of your life are seen to. This can be achieved in how you live your life on a day-to-day basis. We have to work out what is important to us, what gives us joy and ensure that our lives are centred around these things.

Laura Vanderkam, the time management expert, highlights this in her TED talk. She explains that time is highly elastic and it responds to our priorities. Below are some of the points that she goes into:

- When we build the lives we want, time saves itself.

- Time is highly elastic, it responds to our priorities.

- 'I don't have time' means it is not a priority.

- We have the power to fill our lives with what deserves to be there.

Some of Laura Vanderkam's suggestions about how to manage our time are:

- Discover three to five things in your career, relationships and self-care that will make the year amazing.

- Break them down into doable steps then put the steps in your diary.

- Look at the whole of your time and see where the good stuff can go.

- When you actually look at how you spend your time, you will be amazed at how much of it you waste.

I have a very busy life. I am a mother with two businesses. Anyone of these things could be a full-time endeavour on its own. Then, for some bizarre reason, which I can only put down to a midlife crisis, I decided to follow my passion and write a book. Where on earth was I going to find the time? I work seven days a week in the summer months. The plan was to write the book in the winter when my sports management business goes quiet. This was a good plan on paper, but somehow I managed to fritter away my winter months and before I knew it the summer had arrived and I was going full throttle. My editor was waiting for the manuscript and I had already moved the deadline back by a month. I really had to produce the goods. Where was I going to find the time? I get up at 5am at weekends in the summer because of my sports business. I finish work by 9am, but then I will come home, have breakfast with the kids and my husband, and potter about doing nothing in particular. That is normally my free time to catch up on any TV programmes I have recorded during the week. If I have nothing recorded I will go hunting for rubbish to watch to while away the time. If I have a good book on the go, this is also a good reading window. Now that I had to write a book, the pressure was on and I had to find time. Somehow, I managed to set aside four hours every day at the weekend to work on the manuscript. What gave? The recorded TV programmes. What changed? My priorities. Once I got clear on my priorities, I sat in front of the same TV but it remained switched off, while my laptop came on and I typed and researched. From about midday to early evening, everyone knew to leave me alone. If I had gotten my act together in the winter, I would have had more time to play with. There is a saying: 'If you want something to be done, give it to a busy person!' The summer was my busiest time, but it was also when I was at my most productive.

When we get our time management issues sorted out, we eliminate a lot of our stress because we are living a life that is aligned with our values. Our time is spent doing the things that matter and sustain us. Get into the habit of routinely evaluating how you are spending your time. Is your time spent on things that matter to you?

Boundaries

This is a big one for me and anyone who knows me will be surprised that this is an issue. This is because some things are black and white to me and I take no prisoners. When it comes to people in authority or people I view as stronger than me, I am really clear. No one is taking advantage of me, period! Sometimes the balls I have when it comes to standing up for myself and standing up to people in authority astounds me. This is the side of me that colleagues see at work. There is, however, another side. It is really easy for the people I don't believe are as strong as me, or are vulnerable even, to take advantage of me.

You see, I was brought up to be kind to those less fortunate. However, nobody told me that just because they are less fortunate doesn't mean they are good people. This is where my boundary issues reside. The fact is, it is perfectly possible for the disadvantaged to violate your boundaries. They are just being their disadvantaged self and don't know any better. Some of them always look to someone else to take care of them. This activates my saviour complex and before I know it I can't even spell boundary and my life is firmly residing on the back burner while I allow them to run roughshod, albeit in a disadvantaged way, over me.

I have had to work very hard at my split personality when it comes to boundaries. Some of you might be wondering where your boundaries are.

If it makes you feel uncomfortable, chances are your boundaries are being violated.

The aeroplane analogy is a good one for boundaries. You cannot take care of someone until you have taken care of yourself, and this includes the vulnerable and your dependants. In an aeroplane emergency, the advice is to put your oxygen mask on first before your baby's. You are no use to man or beast if you have passed out due to lack of oxygen in an emergency.

Women will give and keep on giving until they have passed out. In my case, I was reaching the pass out point more frequently than was necessary. In the long run this resulted in me standing in a gynaecologist's waiting room and doubting my sanity. For me, a hormone imbalance could not have been a clearer sign that my life was out of balance. I wasn't respecting my own boundaries, never mind not letting other people disregard them. You have to know what serves you. Include this in your priorities and let the people around you know. Remember when we explored nonviolent communication? This can be used in normal conversations, as well as to establish your boundaries. It's an essential part of your self-care. If you think self-care is all about having a massage or a pedicure then think again.

You should know what you can afford to give and stick to it. This should apply to all areas of your life, but it tends to be most evident in your time and money.

Here is another example of doing what is important to you.

I love the idea of volunteering, but with two businesses, two children, a husband and two dogs, I am time poor. I would be doing everyone a disservice if I suddenly decided that I was off to volunteer when half the time when I am not working or seeing to my other duties, I have to fight for time for myself. The fact that something is a good thing to do does not mean that it is a good thing for you to do at this time of your life. This is where time management comes in. If you have worked on your priorities and are clear on them, it is very difficult to allow your boundaries to be violated. I can't volunteer on weekend mornings even in the winter when I am not working. This is because I love to go for walks with my dogs. Sometimes, my younger son decides to come along on his bike too. It is the only time in the week we get to have uninterrupted one-on-one time. He tells me things during the walks we share that he would never tell me otherwise. Anyone with boys knows that it is nigh on impossible to get things out of them. Maybe it is the fact that I am just walking and not asking that makes him open up. Although I think there is something about walking in nature that calms everyone down. This time is protected: a lot of my values are taken care of in that moment. The dogs and I get our exercise and I guess my son gets his exercise too, but the main thing is that my time with him is limited. When he leaves home or decides to stop coming on the walks altogether, like his older brother has, that slot might become available to volunteering (if I move my exercise to another slot), but if I don't protect that time now I will be putting my son at a disadvantage. I will also be missing out on my favourite form of exercise. Without exercise I will become off-kilter and before I know it the stress will set in.

CHAPTER ELEVEN

LET'S TALK ABOUT STRESS, BABY

There is more to life than increasing its speed.

~ MAHATMA GANDHI

Stress

Stress in the emotional sense used to be a noun, but it has seamlessly transitioned into a verb. We are either stressed out or stressing, and half of the time it is over completely avoidable things. Our way of life now almost always has chronic stress baked into it, in one way or another. In a perfect world, we would build our lives devoid of stress, except for what life throws at us that we can't control. This type of stress should keep us stimulated. It is possible to look forward to the unknown because you have got the contingency and capacity to deal with it. This should be exciting, but if you are constantly stressed out, the thought of the unknown leaves you cowering. Your plate is already full so there is no room for the surprises that the universe throws at us to force us to grow. So in our fear we stay stagnated.

You might have heard the saying, 'What doesn't kill you makes you stronger.' Whoever came up with that saying was obviously not dealing with stressed-out individuals. In our world now, it's more like, 'What doesn't kill you puts you on anti-depressants!' One of the titles I thought of for this book was *How to Live Without Prozac!*

The modern malaise of stress is quietly ruining our lives. We insist on living back to front lives, which leads to stress. We are not living in alignment with what matters most to us. We say 'yes' when we should be saying 'no' because we don't even know where our boundaries are. Unfortunately, our bodies know where our boundaries are, so when they are violated we get the stress feedback. There has been study after study about the effects of stress and guess what? It is never good news. A bit of stress can keep us on our toes and helps us grow, but the modern pace of life is such that we are under constant, unremitting stress. That is deadly – literally.

I've personally never understood why we feel the need to pack so much into our lives. Sometimes just hearing other mothers talk at the school gates makes me feel tired. Call me lazy, but I don't think our kids need to be managed within an inch of their lives. They need some time to just potter and get bored. It is supposed to stimulate their creativity. I have also told my kids that it is not my job to keep them entertained. I won't repeat here what I tell them about the people who get bored. Modern parenting has become so competitive, not to mention how kids are overloaded with homework. Plus, us parents have to taxi them around everywhere now because we think every other man they are exposed to other than their dad or teacher is a paedophile! This is crazy. Throw in the fact that we have to work as well, and we find ourselves at our wits' end. Did you know that mothers in the 60s spent 50% less time with their children than mothers in 2012? Intensive parenting is all the rage these days. Not only are our lives crazy but we are also bringing up a generation of over-managed children that expect us to do their bidding. Meanwhile, we are running ourselves ragged.

Don't get me wrong, I am all for parents being engaged with their children and spending time with them. I took my one-year-old on a business trip once, complete with the nanny, because I wanted to stay engaged as my husband was out of the country as well. I am all about being involved.

If both parents work, more often than not it will be the woman who gets home and still has to sort out dinner and get on top of the housework. Most women haven't got the skills to negotiate equality on the home front. This leads to very long days indeed and more stress.

We have the statistics from Chapter 9 to demonstrate the impact of the mother's wellbeing on the long-term happiness of her child. It is three times more than the second highest factor of family income. Rather than intensive parenting for its own sake, it should be balanced parenting, where both parents are involved and the child has some time to him/herself. The mother also gets time to herself and is not working or taking care of someone throughout her waking hours. If the mother is not stressed out, everyone benefits.

Effects of stress

Let's look at the effect of stress on the body, our mood and behaviour. The table below shows the bodily systems affected and how this manifests in disease.

Systems Affected	Effect	Symptoms
Central Nervous and Endocrine System	Fight or flight response	Over/under eating
		Social withdrawal
		Alcohol or drug abuse
Respiratory and Cardiovascular	Heart works too hard	Strokes
		Heart attacks
		Increase in blood pressure
		Strokes
		Heart attacks

Digestive System	Too much glucose	Type 2 diabetes
	Increase in hormones, Rapid breathing, Increase in the heart rate Upset digestive processes	Acid reflux
		Ulcers to flare up
	The way food moves through the body	Diarrhoea
		Constipation
		Nausea
		Vomiting
Muscular System	Constant muscle tensing	Headache
		Backache
		Shoulder pain
Reproductive System	Stress is exhausting for the body and mind	Decrease in the production of testosterone
		Disruption to the woman's monthly cycle
		Heavy/painful periods
		Exacerbate menopause symptoms
Immune System	Weaken the immune system	Flu, colds
		Other infections

Table 4. Effects of Stress

Stress Management

- **Identify your stressors**

  First of all, you must identify your triggers. This forces you to take responsibility. It is hard to manage something you haven't identified.

- **Change what you can**

  You can't eliminate all stress from your life, nor should you want to. You need some stress to feel alive. The trick is to deal with the triggers that are under your control. If being late stresses you out, set your alarm five minutes earlier.

- **Know your limits**

  When they were small, my kids would literally keep running around in the evenings until their legs buckled. They had no idea when they were tired so they kept going. It was quite funny to watch sometimes. I had them in a routine so this falling about didn't happen that often, as I knew when it was time to send them to bed. Don't be like a child. You are a grown woman so know your limits and learn to operate within them. You might think you have the patience of Mother Theresa, but if you are in the second half of your luteal phase and premenstrual, you might find that it's not the best time to offer to have next door's kids over for a play date. Do not ignore the phases of your cycle. Do the intelligent thing and honour your biology. You were built like that for a reason.

- **Involve other people**

  First off, involve your partner! Men have a habit of standing around and not noticing when we need them to do something. You can fight it and add to your stress or you can start spelling things out respectfully. Ask them nicely (I know, I know, why do we even have to ask?) and they will surprise you and halve your stress. They are not being obtuse, they just have 'man brain' and believe it or not, it has its uses in the middle of the night when you think there is an intruder and they go charging down the stairs while you pretend to be part of the duvet. Drop your superwoman act and ask for help. It doesn't have to be just your partner: ask friends, neighbours and frankly anyone who crosses your path who is capable and willing to help. Also, by asking for help, you'll forge closer relationships with people. They'll see that you are only human after all. Closer relationships contribute to our sense of wellbeing, so why not have two for the price of one?

- **Socialise, socialise, socialise**

  I am a social animal. I love having people round and having a chat. I love all things social. Just sitting and chatting to people or listening to other people's problems always makes me feel good about myself. It makes me feel that we all face the same challenges and it gives me a sense of belonging. I promise you that whatever you are going through, you are probably not the first person on earth to have experienced it. Reach out to people and allow them to surprise you.

We are social animals and are built to interact with one another. Loneliness is detrimental to our health. In their studies on loneliness, researchers Julianne Holt-Lunstad, Timothy B. Smith and J. Bradley Layton found how much the following impacted one's odds of dying:

» **Air pollution 5%**

» **Obesity 20%**

» **Excessive drinking 30%**

» **Loneliness 45%**

We are all familiar with how obesity and excessive drinking are bad for us, but no one ever goes on about how loneliness far outstrips them. You need your relationships just as much as you need food. Now chew on that.

Socialise with people you don't know that well. You can't go out with people you barely know and start whingeing about whatever rut you think you are stuck in. This forces you to focus on something else or perhaps shut up while someone else gets a word in edgeways. Remember about taking control and changing your point of focus to what serves you? Socialising with strangers does that for you.

- **Relaxation techniques**

  Mindfulness is all the rage these days. It doesn't matter how you start. Take a yoga or meditation class, do some tai chi or whatever tickles your fancy, but do something along those lines to help you relax. I discuss meditation more in Chapter 14, so stay tuned.

- **Exercise**

  The impact of exercise on stress is immediate. Endorphins are released and suddenly the world doesn't seem like such a scary place after all. It provides you with an outlet. Anyone can go for a run or a brisk walk. There are no barriers to entry but yourself. Put on your trainers and head out. I resisted running for years. I didn't like it and I am still not sure I like it, but when it comes to stress, nothing gets it out of me more than running. I get out there, work up a sweat and come back with endorphins swirling through my body. Suddenly, life feels different. I still prefer a walk to a run any day of the week, as a slower pace allows me to take in the scenery around me, but when I am stressed out, I have to run.

- **Move your point of focus to the positive**

  You cannot suddenly go from the stressed-out person you are now to an optimistic, bright person. But you can change what you are focusing on. You can break the cycle of your thoughts and pull your head out of the funk. I have discussed this already. Your thoughts affect your feelings, so break the cycle. Think about something else. Children are great at pulling you out of your funk and forcing you to focus on a worm they have dug up in the garden. Thank God for small mercies I say.

- **Actively pursue recreation and leisure**

  This is such a life saver. I have taken up gardening and what a pleasure it has been. Find something you enjoy and just go for it with wild abandon. Have fun. Yes, fun. How many of us actually schedule fun into our lives? This should be just as important as the time we schedule in our diary for business meetings. It should not be an afterthought. I have been sitting and staring at my beautiful flowerpot, which is filled with annuals. It really is beautiful and I can feel the stress draining out of my body as I gaze at it. I always used to come last in art class and I am that bad that I seriously cannot draw a straight line with a ruler, but here I am now looking at a flowerpot and wishing I had an easel. What I will do with it is neither here nor there, the point is that I am not focusing on my problems. I am now fancying myself as the next Monet! Surely that is better than stewing in stress.

Recreation and pleasure

I am going to delve into using recreation and pleasure as a combatant to stress. I love to have a good laugh and I love to cook and have people round, but above all, I love to have a good old chinwag. I find people infinitely interesting. Whenever I meet someone for the first time, I want to drag them into a corner and get the story of their life. I have been told I ask too many questions. Watch out for the Spanish Inquisition if you ever meet me. I believe we all process a piece of life's puzzle in our own way and everyone has got a unique perspective. I just love chatting and getting this out of people. I really could chat until the cows came home. But, how many times do I schedule that into my life? OK, so I have done all this work on myself and I know my values and my boundaries, but how many times do I actually schedule the things that I love into my life? Here is what is staggering. I made a conscious effort to schedule dates with my friends whenever I could. That was my New Year's resolution a few years ago. But, believe it or not, most people are too busy being busy to have fun! Yep, not everyone has had their midlife crisis like me and is looking around for a way to live a better life.

My values are still intrinsically linked with the values of others, it seems. It stunned me to realise that during the years of working my socks off I had surrounded myself with people doing the same thing. Life was reduced to snatched conversations at the school gates or the superficial chats in the office, where everyone had a 'perfect' life. To have a real, open conversation with someone these days is like pulling teeth. First of all, you have to schedule a date so far in advance that you forget to look forward to it. Then it pops up in your diary when you are least expecting it, at which point you wonder why you thought dinner in the middle of that week was a good idea in the first place. When you eventually meet up, assuming you haven't had a hard day at work, little Jimmy decided the night before was a good one for teething so you are practically too exhausted to have a decent conversation. Still, you plough on anyway because you had to wait so long for this dinner and you are going to have a good time if it kills you. Did I mention that this is the dinner with your really good friend that you normally have a laugh with? Anyway, eventually you get going. You start with a whinge about the men in your life (it has to be done), then work, then the kids, the extension, the ageing parents. Need I go on? This was supposed to be your fun night with your friend. It is now a whingefest! Are we having fun yet? Still, a problem shared…

I am sure I must come across as desperate sometimes, but I seem to be the only one looking for a good chinwag. I don't have more time than anyone else, I just know that a good laugh with a friend is worth its weight in gold. The research is already there about how our personal relationships have more than twice the positive impact than our pay. We also know that loneliness is more dangerous to us than obesity or excessive drinking. I am sure there will soon be statistics released on the positive impact that going out and having a laugh has on our wellbeing, compared to taking a bunch of vitamins. I have nothing against vitamins, I take them myself, but we would rather pop a pill than do the things that really support our wellbeing. I haven't got empirical evidence yet, but I know it in my innards that at the very minimum, going out for a laugh is just as beneficial as taking anti-depressants. The problem is that our lives are such that we can't go out with our friends and family every night, yet we can pop a pill regularly.

Some people see pleasure and recreation as a luxury or indulgence rather than a need. They can only have fun when they are half naked on a yacht with an entourage. So until said yacht materialises, their enjoyment of life is on hold. Isn't that just crazy? You can have fun and pleasure anywhere. All you need to do is go to an African village where people are dirt poor. In the evenings they will gather in the village centre and have a good old song and dance to the rhythm of beating drums. That is exercise and personal relationships rolled into one. So as long as you are well, all that you need is to make up your mind to have fun.

If you are waiting for your entourage and the yacht, I have got news for you. The money issues and other worries will never go away. They will morph into something else. It is like you are trying for a baby and your only thought is: 'I will be so happy once I have a baby'. What you don't bargain for is the sleepless nights, the tiredness, the sore breasts and the stretch marks that come with having a baby. When we are wishing for something, we see only the positive. Duality is a part of life so there will never be a moment where everything is perfect. Now that you have wrapped your head around that, you might as well have fun now. You have to play like your life depends on it, because it does – only you just don't know it yet.

When you are stressed out and manage to go and have a good laugh, you can literally feel the knots in your shoulders loosening. Children understand the need for play at a basic level. All they want to do is play. We lose that ability as grownups. I know that after a hard day's work in the office battling the next upstart who wants to keep beating their chest and baring their teeth, the last thing you want to do when you get home is jump up and down on the trampoline because little Jimmy wants to. A bottle of wine in front of the telly can seem more appealing, and to be fair it is easier.

Creativity

When I was at school, I won the prize for creativity in my year. My father was at the prize-giving ceremony with his friend, who was a bit hard of hearing and didn't clock what the prize was for. I refused to tell him when he asked because I was ashamed I hadn't won the prize for something in science or maths! At what point in my young life did I decide that science was more valuable than creativity? What in our education system puts creativity at the bottom of the pile when we need both the left and right halves of the brain to live a balanced life and be creative?

What does creativity even mean?

Creativity: The use of imagination or original ideas to create something: inventiveness.

Being creative is more complex than was first thought. We used to think that creativity came from the right side of the brain. Neuroscientists investigating what happens during the creative process have come up with new findings.

Different brain regions are recruited depending on the stage of the creative process, and what you are actually attempting to create. Many of these brain regions work as a team to get the job done, recruiting structures from both the left and right side of the brain.

We are all born creative. Whether we use it is another matter. I have come across people who think they aren't creative. How can anyone think that? If you've got a brain in your head, and by this I mean the grey physical mass, you are creative. To pursue our joy and combat stress we have to deploy our creativity.

When we learn to play as grownups, we allow ourselves to get in touch with the child within. That is where our creativity resides. Our childhood was the part of our lives when we were free from the stresses of having to earn a living – we got to play instead. It was the time when we felt safe enough to be as open as a flower and everything was possible and magical. That point before we took on limitations was when our creativity was allowed to blossom. We weren't closed minded and gave everything a chance.

Creativity allows you to access what you are good at. If you indulge in what you are talented at, you enjoy it and time flies. We will discuss this some more when we get to the work section of this book. I indulge in my creativity when I am cooking or baking. I love to mix different ingredients and try new things. It doesn't always work out, but when it does I feel invigorated. It's such a buzz when people love my inventions and polish off everything on their plates. It is no secret that I am into healthy eating and to most people this is boring and just for people on a diet. So when I have people round and I am able to serve them healthy whole foods that are tasty, it makes me feel good on at least four counts:

1. I am dealing with my personal relationships, which I know is a big contributor to my wellbeing.

2. I am indulging in creativity, which makes me feel clever and keeps my brain cells ticking.

3. My friends are enjoying a good, wholesome and tasty meal.

4. I am helping my friends eat well and contributing to their wellbeing, rather than feeding them processed crap with all the nutrients sucked out of them. (This is a real silent pleasure. A friend once asked me where I got my brown rice mix. This is from someone who existed purely on processed food!)

As grown-ups with all the stresses and strains of modern living, we hardly ever pause to think of creativity. There is a way to access that state of being where we stay open even in the midst of fear and stress. It is called meditation. I will delve into this more in the chapter on spirituality.

CHAPTER TWELVE

THE 3 Rs

I have no special talent. I am passionately curious.

~ ALBERT EINSTEIN

Mental

I am someone who loves knowledge for its own sake. I sometimes wish I could just look at a book and the contents would magically end up in my head. As far as I'm concerned, Kindle and Audible are the best things since sliced bread. I guess I am curious by nature. I don't know where I would be in my life without my habit of life-long learning. When some people are upset, they go for retail therapy and buy clothes and shoes. When I am upset, I go and buy a book. I have been known to phone in sick at work just so I can finish a book!

In Chapter 7, I referred to the Public Health England (PHE) report about dementia and Alzheimer's disease being the biggest cause of death among women. One of the things thought to stave off dementia and Alzheimer's is keeping your brain active by developing new neural networks, i.e. learning new things.

Life-long learning has stood me in very good stead. I have acquired knowledge when I needed it, and it also means I can hold a conversation with just about anyone, as I am interested in a lot of things. For the topics I don't know anything about, I am just as eager to learn and people love it when you listen to them. Add into the mix that I believe everyone has got a story to tell, and it makes new knowledge even more interesting to me. Why am I telling you all this? Because in this day and age, there is no excuse for ignorance. Information is at our fingertips, literally.

My love of reading and life-long learning means I have got a growth mindset. Yep, there is a posh phrase for my condition – growth mindset! Carol Dweck's book, *Mindset: Changing the way you think to fulfil your potential* goes into detail about the growth mindset. Basically, it means you don't believe your abilities are fixed and therefore you can learn anything. You reckon that with effort you can become anything.

I personally think all teachers should be made to buy into this philosophy. I have met teachers who are closed-minded about the children they teach and allow them to think they are not good at certain subjects. To me that is a travesty. Especially as teachers hold such power over the children they teach. No one is 'not good' at anything. Go back and read that sentence again. We have an affinity for certain things and not others, but even with the things that we have affinity for, natural ability will only take you so far. The rest is just sheer hard graft and persistence. What do they say? It takes 10,000 hours to make a genius? Children should be made to understand that with effort they can crack any subject. They should never be allowed to say 'I am not good' at such and such. You might not want to spend the rest of your life cracking calculus, but if you are interested in it and put in the effort, you will crack it. I have crossed many a sword with my children's teachers when they didn't want to take on the fight with me of making the children understand that ability grows with effort. The talent that is wasted simply because children are not encouraged to make the effort makes my blood boil.

Both my sons love swimming, but one of them has a very beautiful stroke. He just glides effortlessly through the water. Everyone comments on it. The interesting thing is, he didn't come by this beautiful stroke by accident. When he was about six, he went swimming with his dad and when his dad wasn't looking he jumped into the deep end of the pool and gave himself and everyone else a fright. He then developed a phobia of swimming and decided it wasn't for him. Meanwhile, my husband was too traumatised to take him for swimming lessons. Luckily for me, I wasn't there when the incident took place and was spared the trauma. Both my husband and I agreed that swimming was a life skill so he couldn't give up on it. I took him to a couple of group swimming lessons, but he screamed his way through them, which proved disruptive for the other kids. I was told by the swimming instructor to pursue other avenues, as the other parents were complaining. I took him down the one-to-one swimming lesson route, which was expensive, but I couldn't afford to give up and have him sit at the edge of the pool for family holidays. (I guess I should have focused on the life skill part, but I didn't want to be babysitting a child on family holidays when I would rather they be off with their dad so I could enjoy my hard-earned time alone on the beach with a good book.) I found him a personal swimming instructor and I also bribed, I mean rewarded, him with computer games whenever he didn't scream and went calmly into the water.

He started off in the toddler pool, which was full of urine and screaming toddlers, and he soon realised that he was too big for that nonsense. That spurred him on to get his act together. No one wants to learn to put their face in the water in a pool full of other kids' urine, so he quickly graduated to the main pool. Once he felt comfortable enough to get his face wet, we were away. His swimming got better and better and eventually he was able to go back into a mainstream class without screaming the house down. His beautiful stroke is the result of the one-to-one lessons he had. He is 17 now and doesn't even remember having a phobia about swimming. What is the point of this story? The growth mindset! I couldn't afford to give up so we persevered and now we have a beautiful, confident swimmer.

I believe you can improve at anything, even the things that you don't like and that frighten you to death. Nothing is set in stone. You choose whatever you want to learn or become and go for it. The fact that you might not have been good at it in the past is neither here nor there. If you are genuinely interested in it now, be prepared to put in the effort – even if that involves putting your face in a pool full of toddlers' urine – and you will acquire the skills you need to become whatever you want to become.

The thing is, you tend to try harder at the things you like, so it is easier to make the 10,000-hours mark without feeling like your teeth are going to fall out. I believe children should be aligned with what they love, and then be made to make the effort until they realise how great they are at it. That is where they will find their confidence, because it is linked with the effort.

Just being good at something without knowing why doesn't make you confident about your ability. However, when you have consciously put in the effort, had some obstacles thrown in and you have overcome them, you will know you are solid in that ability and no one can take it away from you.

I have applied life-long learning to staying healthy. Women say to me all the time, 'It is alright for you, you are naturally slim.' I always roll my eyes at this. OK, so I was like a stick insect when I was a teenager and one of the last people to have a period in my year group. I also had to stuff my bra with tissues because my body was playing catch-up and all the other girls had breasts. That said, no one who has had children and has gone through the vagaries of what your body and hormones put you through is naturally slim. I may have had the build of a slim person when I was young, but lots of girls I started out with had the same build and no longer look anything like me. I am not saying this to be boastful. I am saying this to prove that I have spent a long time learning about how to support my body and be healthy. My weight, therefore, has taken care of itself. I have learnt about what to eat, how to exercise and how to respect the phases of my cycle. The result is good health. As far as I am concerned, you cannot afford to be alive and not learn.

In this modern world, things change all the time. In 1965, Gordon Moore, who became one of the founders of Intel, the computer chip making company, wrote a paper that later became known as Moore's law. The premise was that computing power would double every year. In 1971, this was revised to every two years.

His predictions have held out. In technology, the gadgets that we were using three years ago are already obsolete. We now change our phones every 18-months and every time we get a new one, it comes packed with more features than we know what to do with. My phone is now the remote control for my TV! I was shocked the other day when I couldn't start my car with my phone. This is how high my expectations now are, but I bet by the time this book comes out starting your car with your phone will be routine.

My children show me things all the time on their phone that make my eyeballs revolve in my head. New technology is coming out at the rate of knots. You can't even go to the dentist these days without being confronted with some new-fangled way of updating your medical history on a hand-held device. You cannot afford to have a fixed mindset and not feel challenged by life. In order to be able to go with the flow and not feel stressed out by all the changes within modern living, you have to be prepared to learn something new every day.

In his TED talk, The Learning Expert, Eduardo Briceño explains about learning and performance. He says there is a learning zone and a performance zone and most grown-ups spend their time in the performance zone.

If you think about it, we learn what we have to learn at college or university, or on-the-job training. But once we start performing, we get stuck in that zone. This means we perform at the same level forever. If we want to increase our performance, then we need to take time out, go back to the learning zone and learn new skills. Therein lies the problem. As children we are allowed to make mistakes and no one judges us. As grown-ups, it's quite a different kettle of fish. For starters your self-talk (AKA the voice in your head) will not let you off the hook if you make a mistake. This is when we have to make the space and the time to go back to the learning zone in a safe environment. We can learn and practice and then come back to the performance zone to perform.

If there is something you have always wanted to learn how to do, make the time and go and learn it. Go and fall flat on your face in a safe environment, then practice until you are competent before returning to the performance zone. Make this a lifestyle choice. Add something to your skills every year.

I am adding gardening to my life skills this year. I have got a big garden, which was mainly laid to lawn. My neighbours had been hinting about what a waste it was. This fell on deaf ears because my husband and I didn't see ourselves as gardeners. We had a gardener who came once a fortnight and did something (don't ask me what), but so far as the grass was cut and the garden looked nice enough, I was fine with it. (The gardener was a young, ripped lad with long blond hair in a ponytail. I am no Lady Chatterley, but there is nothing wrong with admiring nature, and I am not talking about the garden!) I did dabble with a herb garden every now and then. I love the idea of eating fresh herbs from my own garden, but I must admit they mainly came from the supermarket. The gardener, bless him, tended to my herb garden and tried his best to decipher the herbs from the weeds.

This year, we are doing up the house and so we decided to have the garden designed properly. Then we'd have a proper grownup house and a garden to match. For starters, I had no idea how much digging was going to be involved or how many wheelbarrows of earth had to be moved from one part of the garden to the other. I had no clue how much trees and shrubs cost or how much watering I'd have to get up and do in the morning before work. The annuals in the pot that inspired me to bring out the easel have to be watered twice a day…before the sun comes up and after it goes down. At the risk of trivialising the Nobel institution, I think the person who invented the sprinkler should be given a prize! There is something rather mesmerising about sitting on the patio and watching the sprinkler go from side to side. Maybe I should get out more, but I love to watch the sprinkler. Anyway, to cut a long story short, I had no idea what gardening entailed.

One of our neighbours, who has the most beautiful cottage garden and has won 'Garden of the Year' in our village for two years in a row, is designing our garden. He has got his work cut out taking on two gardening reprobates. My husband and I are convinced he is squatting in our shed, as he seems to pop up out of nowhere every time we go near the garden, just to tell us how we are doing it all wrong. We had the flowerbed rotivated (yep, it is a word and I hadn't heard of it before, either) but he, the neighbour that is, decided there were too many roots in the soil after said rotivating. So we had to go and dig to get all the roots out. We live in a part of Hertfordshire which was occupied by Romans. I am convinced half their living quarters are buried under our garden. You cannot dig without hitting a rock, a piece of pottery, a horseshoe or something else of that ilk. The dogs looked on (the dogs look on a lot and I have got a lingering resentment towards them) while my husband, the kids and I dug the bed and did our best to take all the roots out. Then the aforementioned neighbour/garden designer popped out of the shed again. I kid you not, he said we had done it all wrong. We had trampled on the soil while digging, therefore stopping it from breathing. That's not all. We hadn't dug deep enough and so we had to do it all over again. Just to rub salt into our wounds, he gave us a demonstration on how to do it properly. I am not being funny here, but wasn't that locking the barn door after the horse had bolted? Wasn't the demo needed before we spent two hours digging the wrong way? You know when you are halfway through something and you start thinking, 'this was just a bad idea'? Where was my ribbed, blond gardener when I needed one? Just to give you some context, I hadn't done any digging since I was a child. Even then, the digging I did was for fun and worms. Nothing strenuous there. Now here I was being asked to dig soil that had half the Roman civilisation buried underneath it.

Did I really know what I was taking on with this gardening malarkey?

NO. I had no idea how many headlocks I was going to get into with the shrubs while being sprayed with water from the sprinkler, which was just doing its thing.

Am I glad I am doing it?

Ask me again in six months.

Am I in the learning zone?

I'm firmly planted (pardon the pun) in it.

Am I learning new skills?

Where do I start? Well, I know my Gleditsia from my Helleborus. It is more physical than I ever anticipated so I am getting a proper workout with all the squats, lifting, bending and twisting. Not only am I going to get a good-looking garden, I will be well toned at the end of it all. So, what's not to like? Plus, I will now be able to impress people with my knowledge of plants, especially when I start rattling off the Latin names. I'll also be staving off dementia while I'm at it.

While I have been in the learning zone with the gardening, there has been no judgement. It is a safe place for me to fall in the mud over the wheelbarrow with half a shrub attached to my hair. You need that abandon to learn new skills and invigorate your life.

Indeed, throughout life, we have to alternate between the learning and performance zones. Tell you what, it would be really neat if we could replicate that in the different areas of our lives as well. Let's go onto work.

CHAPTER THIRTEEN

YOUR WORK OR YOUR LIFE!

*Your work is going to fill a large part of your life, and the only way
to be truly satisfied is to do what you believe is great work.
And the only way to do great work is to love what you do.
If you haven't found it yet, keep looking. Don't settle. As with all
matters of the heart, you'll know when you find it.*

~ STEVE JOBS

We now know all about the performance zone, so where do we operate most in the performance zone? Work. Work is an interesting place. We spend a lot of our waking hours there, but it is also the place where we're the most hesitant to be ourselves. There are overt and covert parameters for us to operate within, and in some workplaces you can spend a lifetime trying to decipher the behavioural codes.

Do you remember when you were the fresh-faced work experience kid doing all the fetching and carrying and your best friend seemed to be the photocopier? Now that you are grown up, and you are a fully-fledged woman juggling several balls, only one of them happens to be work. So how is it going? Are you constantly looking over your shoulder at the next generation of girls yapping at your heels? Do you find you say something in a meeting and it seems to go unheard, while a male colleague says the same thing and suddenly there are nods all around? How did you cope with pregnancy at work? Were you patronised within an inch of your life because someone got it into their heads that pregnant women can't pull off a high-powered meeting? My personal favourite was coming back to work after giving birth.

I took six months' maternity leave for my first baby. Everything went swimmingly until the day I was due back at work. The baby, who by now was beginning to get mobile, decided this was the best day to fall off the bed! After six months off, I couldn't phone in and say, 'I forgot to have eyes put in the back of my head and as a consequence my baby fell off the bed and now I am taking him to see the doctor just in case he has a brain injury.' I left him with my mother with a long list of instructions and went to work. I phoned her every hour, on the hour, to see if he was still alive, how his breathing and movements were and what his temperature was. My poor mum was driven to distraction. She had brought up six children of her own, so you would have thought she would know if a baby wasn't breathing.

I was still breastfeeding at this point and in my panic to get to work on time, I forgot to use my breast pads. Lunchtime found me in the toilets fashioning breast pads out of toilet roll and wondering how long they would last before I started leaking into my top. In between phone calls to my mum and breast pad watch, I still had to attend several meetings and, as it was my first day back, I had to chirrup about how happy I was to have returned to the fold. I was damned if I was going to let anyone think that childbirth had watered down my intellectual capacity or my ambition. I had a point to prove, which was that I was just as capable as I was before I left.

By the end of the day, I was completely exhausted, both physically and emotionally. I remember sitting in the car in the car park, by which point my homemade breast pads had finally caved into the pressure of my engorged breasts and I had started leaking. I suddenly felt completely overwhelmed and it was only Monday. How was I going to get through the week? I pulled myself together and tackled the one-and-a-half hour commute home. The baby had been fed and bathed by the time I got home and was ready for bed. He wasn't hungry and could hardly keep his eyes open, but my breasts were about to explode, and breast is best, damn it! Of course, this was all for purely selfish reasons. I had missed my baby and needed a cuddle and I also needed the physical release from the build-up of breast milk. After a hard day at work, I was not going to strap myself to a breast pump and feel like a cow to boot. Compare that to what my male colleagues, even the new fathers, probably did that evening when they got home. It's definitely not a level playing field.

I can completely understand why some women just jack it in and become stay-at-home mothers. Not that this is the easy option, either. I would have given up, given half the chance, but my ladder was leaning against the wrong wall. This meant I was not quite living my own life and had bought into a lifestyle that demanded that both parents work.

To add insult to injury, shortly after I came back from maternity leave, I was made redundant. I am no longer bitter about this, honest. It was a blessing in disguise, as I got the chance to really evaluate my life and make different choices, but I didn't see it this way at the time. I was a professional woman and work was part of my self-esteem. Without it I wasn't sure what I was going to talk about at dinner parties or, for that matter, how I was going to describe myself. I had defined myself by what I did for too long.

Interestingly, these days I prefer to talk about gardening. Back then I had spent a lifetime trotting out my 'achievements' at work to the: 'What do you do for a living?' question that is often asked at parties. What was I going to say when suddenly my 'achievements' were just getting through the day without collapsing into an exhausted heap on the bathroom floor with nothing to show for it? Well, nothing except happy, well cared for children.

Unfortunately, there is no business jargon to describe that all-consuming activity called childcare. There is nothing to show for it because it is taken for granted. Women do it day in, day out, and if you are lucky, you get some recognition occasionally.

One time my husband, a human rights lawyer, was due to get an award for his work. I turned up, as any dutiful, proud wife would. The awards were being held in some swanky City of London law firm's offices. I got chatting to one of the organisers. I mentioned how tired I was and she was surprised, as she'd assumed I was a 'lady of leisure'.

Nothing wrong with that, but why is it that some people assume that professionally successful men have to have a stay-at-home wife? Why can't people see that you can have an equally professionally successful woman beside a man, and that it's not always all about the man?

Incidentally, I was tired because I had been up half the night trying to bring up one of the critical IT systems for an oil company before pumps started to run dry at petrol stations the next morning! The saying, 'Behind every successful man there is a woman' is a lot of the time interpreted as a stay-at-home wife. I once saw a bumper sticker that said, 'Behind every successful woman is a pile of ironing.' That really made me smile. I would like to add my own saying here – 'Behind every successful woman is a nanny, a cleaner and a good helping of anti-depressants.' What was the ratio of women on anti-depressants and anxiety medicines again? One in three. If you ask me, success here is only being used in the professional/material sense.

Of course, it doesn't help that there seems to be this rift between women who work outside the home and women who work in the home. I have done both and can see both sides of the argument. This rift would not exist if women who worked inside the home were given their proper due and recognition. The women who go out to work achieve validation in the form of money, status and promotions, etc. The women who work inside the home are mainly ignored. If they are lucky they get to be patronised by the professional types when they get all dolled up to stand by their man. They are seen as the 'little' women who exist just to make their husband and children happy. They are a facilitator and no one asks them about their ambitions and plans for the next five years because they are seen as more of the same.

Putting the monetary aspect aside, these women are making a huge contribution to the stability of society. Apart from their families, they are the ones who normally organise school fairs, assist with reading in primary schools and generally help the school system keep operating with a lot of free labour. If all of them headed out to work outside the home, what would happen? We live in a society that operates on the market economy and puts a value on things based on demand and supply rather than whether it is filling a need. There is an adequate supply of mothers, so it will never be the case that we'd have to pay them. As a consequence, such an important contribution to society goes under the radar.

In 2011, *Forbes* magazine printed an article based on a survey by salary.com saying why stay-at-home mums should earn $115,000 per annum (which is about £88,000 per year). I was thrilled to bits that a leading source for reliable business news and financial information had gone to the trouble of publishing this. Motherhood has always been hard work, but it's also been taken for granted. Finally, someone was giving it the profile it deserves. To arrive at the valuation, motherly duties were broken down into the following aspects:

- Day care centre
- Teacher
- CEO
- Psychologist
- Cook
- Housekeeper
- Laundry machine operator
- Computer operator
- Facilities manager
- Janitor
- Van driver

The survey also stated that stay-at-home mothers typically work a 97-hour week. For those of you reading this who recruit people as part of your role at work, you will see how it would be nigh on impossible to recruit one person with the above skillset, not to mention that no one would be prepared to work a 97-hour week!

I think they left out Personal Assistant (PA), so they should add another £15,000 at least. These days, looking after children involves responding to a multitude of emails from schools, general administrative duties and managing calendars for school trips, play dates and sleepovers. Modern parenting is a labour intensive business.

As already mentioned, according to a study by the University of California, parents in most Western countries today spend more time with their kids than they did in the 1960s. Interestingly, the more educated the parents were, i.e. the professional classes, the more time they spent with their children.

Now that we know the monetary value of staying at home and looking after kids, how many of us can get past our self-esteem and have the balls to go for a £88k job after a five-year career break to look after children? Even if we somehow stumbled past the salary, if the job specification stated the skillsets required were those listed on the previous page, most of us would balk at it.

The truth is, we do an £88k job day in, day out, without even batting an eye. However, without social validation and valuation, we tend to discount it. What we need is a good spin doctor, I mean marketing expert, to work their magic at updating our CV after we have been off work looking after children. They need to make it include all the skills listed so that we can waltz into an £88k role. Seriously, though, if you knew that after maternity leave your skills would be valued at £88k, don't you think that how you felt about yourself after taking time out would be vastly different? Would you make different choices perhaps?

One of my regrets in life is not starting my family five years earlier than I did. I had my mum on my back to start one after I got married. Who listens to their mum anyway? What did she know? Her generation lived for their husbands and children. This was a different generation. We had the pill and we had our careers to think about. I didn't start my family because I wanted my career to be established to the point where I would feel secure enough to take the time off and come back to the same position. For women between the ages of 25 and 30, it is thought that every year away from their career costs £10,000 per annum in pay increases. So I delayed for five years and climbed the greasy pole, only to be made redundant after coming back from maternity leave. Did I say I had let go of the bitterness? Well, it seeps out when I am not looking! Biologically speaking, the best age for women to have children is between 23 and 29.5 years old. I didn't have my first until I was 32. Normally what will hold most women back is the lack of a suitable partner, but even though I had bagged myself a husband, I was chasing the money and the lifestyle.

I personally think taking time out to have kids should be treated, at the very least, the same as taking time out to do a master's degree. In fact, how many women give up altogether after taking time off to raise their children because they have lost their confidence? They feel technology has changed too much and they will not be able to adjust. They may worry there would be too much juggling involved, not to mention that their work suits don't fit anymore.

Data from the Office for National Statistics in the UK suggests that in 2013 there was an increase of 53% in the number of women in work compared with 1971, some 42 years earlier. For men during the same period, there was actually a decrease of 16%. In the US in 2010, the bulk of the labour force was made up of women.

In 1970, between 2% and 4% of women contributed to the family income. Now 40% of them do. Women are now a force to be reckoned with in the workplace. Something really interesting is happening and the trend is only set to continue. So what is society and the government doing to support women in the workplace and ensure they don't abandon ship if they don't want to?

In her brilliant 2010 article 'The End of Men' for The Atlantic magazine, Hanna Rosin argued that for every two BA degrees handed to men, women got three. Additionally, of the 15 categories of jobs where vacancies are expected to increase in the next decade, all but two – janitor and computer engineer – are primarily carried out by women.

In 2010, according to the Bureau of Labor Statistics in the US, 51.4% of managerial and professional jobs were held by women. This was up from 26.1% in 1980. In 2013, across Europe, when looking at top-level senior management roles, which are a step up from normal managerial roles, the figure is still an impressive 33%, with the UK edging ahead of the European average with 35%.

When it comes to intellectual capacity, women and men can now go toe-to-toe, and this is beginning to be reflected in the new white-collar economy. The dog-eat-dog corporate world is changing and it's no longer just about intellectual prowess and leading by might and intimidation, but rather emotional intelligence and soft skills such as collaboration and communication skills. Women tend to have these in spades. I believe that the balance will gradually begin to tilt in favour of women, even in the top managerial roles. But we are still not out of the woods.

The fact still remains that in the UK, according to data from the Office for National Statistics in 2013:

- Above the age of 22, men have consistently higher employment rates than women.
- More men than women tend to work in the professional occupations associated with higher levels of pay.
- Women dominate employment within caring and leisure occupations, which are not the best paid.
- Female graduates are more likely to work in slightly lower-skilled occupation groups than men.
- Men make up the majority of workers in the top 10% of earners for all employees. The good news is that the gap is lower for those under 30.

Call me an optimist and a flag waver for women, but I am really proud to be a woman of this generation. The bra burning our mothers carried out didn't go to waste. But – and there is always a but – while we are making strides in the corporate world, the pile of ironing is still there. At the very minimum, we are expected to look for someone to deal with housework and childcare if we are not going to do it ourselves. This is where we have to be careful.

Now that we have fought our way into the boardroom and men are being challenged to take us seriously, how are we going to ensure that we don't collapse in a heap in the car park with leaky breasts just to prove a point?

Success at work

Do what you love

To be successful at work, for those of us that choose to work outside the home, we have to be doing what we love. I actually don't know that many people who do what they love for a living. I know a lot of people who are doing what they have to do and then do what they love in their spare time.

For those of you still young enough to do a career switch, please, please go after what you love. You will be doing it for a long time and it will take a lot out of you. If you are only doing it for the money you will resent it after a while. Those of you who've taken a career break to look after your children, if you decide to go back, please pause for a minute before you blindly go back to where you left off. This is your chance to pick up something you love and do it for a living.

Hopefully, if you have been able to stay away from work for a few years, you can take the financial risk of starting in a different direction.

"You can only become truly accomplished at something you love. Don't make money your goal. Instead, pursue the things you love doing, and then do them so well that people can't take their eyes off you."

\- MAYA ANGELOU

Get help!

I must say, I never understood the middle-class obsession of doing everything yourself when it comes to childcare. Perhaps this is because I grew up in Africa, where some middle-class women will have a nanny for every child. Even for the working-class women who can't afford nannies, child rearing is never a one-woman job. The whole village steps in. Here in England, if you are not looking after your children yourself, in certain circles you have to be apologetic about it.

Not everyone is cut out to be an Earth Mother. Staying at home and looking after children does not make you noble. A lot of women go out to work out of financial necessity. No one should be made to feel ashamed of the childcare choices they make. If women took the pressure off themselves to be the primary carer and instead took an objective decision about what worked for them, the rift between working and stay-at-home mums would disappear. There would be no need for anyone to give anyone daggers at the school gates.

Doing what works for you means getting in someone to do the bits you don't like, are not good at or are not capable of doing. There is no shame in getting help, be it for the housework or the childcare. We all love our children, but not being with them 24/7 doesn't diminish your love for them in any way. It actually helps them learn to have good relationships with other people, and this goes a long way towards their emotional development.

Once, after the kids in my son's class had come back from a school trip, one mother told me that her son had been very homesick and had cried a lot. Now, my second son tends to be a bit shy, but I still couldn't imagine him being homesick on a school trip. In fact, he had a whale of a time and the teachers saw a whole new and adventurous side to him. My children are very independent. They have had to be, as I have always worked outside the home and they have had to get used to other carers apart from me. The moral of the story is: free yourself from whatever middle-class pressure you are putting yourself under and get help.

Whatever you do, get your husband involved right from day one of your child entering this world. I learnt my lesson the hard way. After being hospitalised after having my second baby, I came home after 10 days to find that my other son had been going to school in the wrong uniform. He had progressed from nursery to year one, where they didn't wear jogging bottoms to school anymore. Instead they sported proper grey trousers. My husband only knew of the old nursery jogging bottoms, so that is what our lad had been dressed in. His teacher later told me that they knew I was in hospital so they excused the oversight.

Don't get me wrong, my husband is the most supportive husband on earth, and he was changing nappies from day one, but he was as involved as I let him be. I had done the school uniform shopping without him and stashed it away so he was none the wiser. So long as I insisted on doing my superwoman bit; holding down a full-time job and managing all the kids' stuff in full-on Earth Mother-mode, he was happy to play with them and do all the fun stuff. Women resent this, but we somehow fail to articulate our needs on the childcare front to the men in our lives.

This might be a good time to go back to the tips I gave you in Chapter 9 on how to communicate your needs. Research from Norway showed that men who take paternity leave are 50% more likely to help around the house for the rest of their lives. If you want to reduce the stress in your life, take the pressure off yourself and get your husband involved. Admittedly, his way of doing things might not quite be up to your standards at the start, but it'll be better by the second child.

Self-care

This is huge if you are working outside the home, because you will be time poor and when you are home you will either be exhausted or feel you have to spend quality time with the kids. Taking time out for yourself can seem like a selfish act. You have been away from home all day so you feel the need to compensate for it. This is faulty thinking.

You need to carve time out for yourself. Remember the oxygen mask on the aeroplane analogy? You have two responsibilities; your family and yourself. Both are of equal importance. You need the most support in the first part of your follicular phase. Let your partner know what is going on so you can buy some time to withdraw. Let him do the bedtime routine so you can put your feet up.

If you aren't looking after yourself, your work will suffer. You need to make sure you are taking care of all your physical needs. Eat well, sleep well, hydrate, exercise and take time out for a pedicure and a massage. You know it makes sense. We are living in the era of the yummy mummy, so being a mother is no longer an excuse to look frumpy and out of shape. You also have to look sharp for the office. You have fought hard for recognition in the boardroom and now you can sashay in with style.

Time management

We discussed this in Chapter 9, so please go and refresh, but as a working mother who wants to be successful, you have to be really hot on your time management. Do not allow other people to waste your time. Here are a few additional tips:

- **Wake up early and get ahead of your day.**
- **Earn your credits as quickly as possible at work.**

  As a working mother, sometimes you will have to let people down. You can't lead that workshop because your child has been running a fever all night and you just can't risk leaving them with the child minder. This is where you need your credits, and by this I mean goodwill. If you have been a good, hardworking employee, then on the odd chance that you have to let people down, your boss will know that it is out of character and cut you some slack. Get to work at earning these credits as soon as you start a new job. Work hard, deliver on time and be true to your word. The time will come when you will literally be coasting on those credits, but you have to earn them first. I simply like to do a good job, so I don't even see it as earning credits, but it sure does pay off.

- **Learn to compartmentalise.**

  If you are at work, you are at work, if you are at home, you are at home. Do not let those boundaries bleed into each other. One work colleague was really surprised when he visited me at home and saw me in full-on mother mode. He only knew me in the work 'take no prisoners, kick arse' mode. Risk being mumsy at work at your peril. Women are still battling stereotypes.

- **Learn to say 'no'.**

  No, you cannot put that last minute PowerPoint presentation together because you have to be at the parent teacher evening. Next time, if you are given enough notice, you will definitely make sure it is ready. If you have earned your credits as per my earlier point, you will also feel more confident about saying no because the powers that be will know you don't take the piss.

- **Be a planner.**

  As a working mum, if you don't plan the wheels will come off the wagon. The juggling simply won't be possible without planning. These days, there is no excuse for forgetting stuff. Your phone is with you at all times, so just put everything on it, set a reminder and be done with it.

- **Learn to be flexible.**

  With all the planning, sometimes you just have to drop everything and go and pick up a child because the school nurse has had enough. During those times, you just have to give an assistant the opportunity to step up while you go and take care of your other business.

- **Meditate (more on this in the next chapter).**

We must not allow ourselves to forget why we are working. British philosopher John Stuart Mill argued that the best use of more wealth is more leisure. You are working and making more money. Don't forget to use it in the best way. Most of us erroneously go for more consumption – the more conspicuous the better. After all, it is a status symbol. Our self-esteem is firmly wrapped up in our consumption. This is a shame, as it leads to more stress.

More affluence should mean more time to spend on activities that contribute the most to our wellbeing, such as close personal relationships. Spending time with our close friends and family is the important stuff, the location and how this happens is just incidental. A holiday in a caravan park in the rain with people that make you feel good is better than one in Saint-Tropez on a yacht with people you care very little about and have to spend half the time pretending to be someone you are not.

And finally...guilt

I can't write a chapter about women and work and not talk about guilt. For a start, parenthood is riddled with guilt, as people tend to blame their parents for all their psychological issues. Add the working mother into the cocktail and the guilt levels go off the chart. We blame ourselves for forgetting about the non-uniform day when our child is the only one who turns up in uniform. (I always told my children not to be afraid to be different, hopefully that dealt with that. It might have created another issue, though, as one of my boys, now that he is the same height as me, thinks nothing of wearing my jogging bottoms to the gym, complete with flared bottoms!)

We feel guilty if the email comes home about forgotten homework. We feel guilty about paying someone else to look after our children. We feel guilty about being tired when we get home. We feel guilty when we have to go on a business trip. We feel guilty when our child is sick and we can't take that day off work. We feel guilty when we can't be there for the Mother's Day school assembly. We feel guilty when we can't be there on sports day to watch him come last in the 100m sprint. You can drive yourself demented with the guilt.

Working mothers' guilt can be debilitating. You feel like you are a jack-of-all-trades and a master of none. I am not quite sure why we feel the need to beat ourselves up about working, but first remind yourself of why you work. For a lot of us, it simply isn't a choice, but even if that wasn't the case, I'm not sure why we should have to justify our decision to anyone. To work or not to work is a personal choice. When you make the choice to work, please, I am begging you, take the pressure off yourself and accept that you will drop the ball every now and then. Have strategies in place to cope with those moments.

Accept that you will always be a bit of an outsider at the school gates and will not be in the midst of all that is going on. That is the price to pay, but you can't have everything and nor should you want everything. Make some good friends with the other mums and let them keep you in the know. Accept that your nanny in some instances will know more about the minutiae of your children's lives than you do, but you will know about the important stuff. Think about it as a shared responsibility. It is a sisterhood, after all, and not a competition.

If you feel judged by your nanny, you have the wrong nanny. In as much as there is research out there showing that working outside the home affects your child, there is just as much suggesting the opposite. Just do what works for you and ditch the guilt. It is an unnecessary accessory.

CHAPTER FOURTEEN

THE GODDESS WITHIN

To enjoy good health, to bring true happiness to one's family, to bring peace to all, one must first discipline and control one's own mind. If a man can control his mind he can find the way to Enlightenment, and all wisdom and virtue will naturally come to him.

~ BUDDHA

Spiritual

If I am being totally honest, this chapter is the main reason why I wanted to write this book. This is my real indulgence. This is the stuff that gets me out of bed. I couldn't wait to get to it. Amazingly, spirituality is now becoming somewhat mainstream and there are aspects of it that are now de rigueur in the corporate world. These days, mindfulness is an everyday word. Go back 20 years and you had to scour occult bookshops to see this kind of stuff. Hit the bookshops that line Charing Cross Road in London today, and you can buy books on the subject by the foot. I remember going into one of the occult shops and it was just me, a couple of hippies and one weirdo browsing the shelves. A few years later, Mind, Body and Spirit sections started to pop up in bookshops like Waterstones.

Luckily, we have got to the part of our evolution in the Western world where people are beginning to realise that happiness does not come from what we own. It comes from who we are. Our economies are rich enough to afford us the lifestyle that prevents us from hiding behind the thought of 'If only I could afford...I would be happy.'

Enough of us can afford it, yet it has not increased our happiness levels. In fact, in some cases, what we have striven for materially has become a burden and added to our stress levels.

How many of us are living a life aligned with our purpose? How many of us have even stopped to ask:

What is my purpose?

Why was I put on this earth?

What sets me on fire?

How can I make a difference?

What can I contribute to the greater good?

Life's purpose/meaning

Don't worry, I am not about to go all religious on you. You have stuck with me this far, so hang on in there. We are going to talk about God, but not in the religious sense. God means a lot of things to a lot of people. The last I heard, God's gender was up for debate. I don't care about the gender of God because God is beyond all that. Some people prefer to use terms like The Universe, Divine Being, The Higher Self, Divine Mother, Cosmic Consciousness…the list is indeed endless.

My idea of God is more aligned with the Higher Self/Divine Consciousness concept. There is a school of thought that says that our highest purpose on this earth is to know God. Now what does that even mean? If your highest purpose is to know your highest self, then suddenly 'God' has got nothing to do with religion. It is about you developing yourself to become the best version of you that you can be.

Here are a few concepts that have helped me:

- We are part of something bigger than ourselves.
- We are part of the whole and we are all connected on some level: animal, mineral and vegetable.

- There is a universal wisdom that we can all tap into for guidance.
- The extent of our spiritual growth is up to us.
- We are all equal in the eyes of the divine and we are all loved.

You don't have to agree with me on these beliefs, you just have to be open minded enough to hear me out. I want to make the case for having a spiritual life, and it starts with meditation.

Getting up early in the morning to meditate is no one's idea of fun, especially in the winter months. Spending more time pressing the snooze button on your alarm could really become an Olympic sport in some circles. That is why I am making the effort to explain to you why you need meditation in your life. Once you understand the need, hopefully you will make the effort. And let's face it, it is an effort in the beginning. Meditation, like any life skill, has got to be learned in the learning zone.

Allow me to throw some science at you, as it really helps the logical, evidence-based people like me to give up our sleep in the mornings. By the way, I really envy those people who can just accept things because someone in authority, such as a guru, looked at them sagely and said, 'Just do it.'

Unfortunately for me, no matter how sage and fast-worn someone looks, whatever they ask me to do has to make sense. Therein lies the downfall of a lot of us in the West. We need PowerPoint slides, charts and figures before we take the leap. This is good and bad at the same time. With things like meditation, for example, you need to take the leap of faith to experience the benefits.

The truth is, most people don't see any results when they start meditating. On the surface, it may seem like nothing is happening so they give up. The hype around meditation also doesn't help. People make a song and dance about it so when you start and you can't hear the song or see the dance it is quite easy to pack it in, especially when you keep falling asleep every time you try to meditate. Believe me when I tell you that I have been at this game for years. I have tried all sorts of techniques, given up and then picked it up again. On and on it goes.

Unfortunately, no one can learn this skill for you, but learn it you must in order to gain peace of mind and the ability to enjoy your life. The more you meditate, the more you will get out of it and the more things will start making sense to you. The more you will realise that a peaceful attitude is the only way forward. Unfortunately, a lot of us are only driven to make the effort when we are in pain, have suffered a loss or feel lost.

By ignoble whips of pain, man is driven at last into the Infinite Presence, whose beauty alone should lure him.

AUTOBIOGRAPHY OF A YOGI – PARAMAHANSA YOGANANDA

Benefits of meditation

There have been tonnes of studies on meditation so we can now evaluate its benefits objectively, with MRI scans or EEG tests, rather than depending on the word of some white-bearded sage in the Himalayas. Below are some of the benefits:

1. **It slows down the ageing of the brain**

   The results of a University of California study in 2015 on meditation concluded that: 'Meditation is brain-protective and associated with a reduced age-related tissue decline.'

   This is indeed good news, especially as we are now aware that Alzheimer's and dementia are the biggest causes of death among women.

2. **It reduces activity in the brain, which in turn reduces worrying**

   This is a big one for me. I was a born worrier. I worry and then I worry about worrying. I wish I were one of those laid-back people who just let things wash over them. I got into meditation for lots of reasons and this was one of the main ones. I was once off work for a year, with no income coming in, and this was an extremely worrying time. Incidentally, this also meant I had time on my hands. I got disciplined and ensured I meditated every day for an hour. After a while, I noticed that I wasn't as reactive to things and I could somehow distance myself from the worrying. It didn't go away, but it didn't control me so much. I could somehow ride the wave.

3. **Meditation has the same effect on depression and anxiety as an anti-depressant**

This was the outcome of a study at John Hopkins University in Baltimore, in 2014.

If you're wondering why people still take anti-depressants and suffer all the associated side effects, I'll tell you. No pharmaceutical company has yet come up with glossy literature about meditation.

Another reason is that popping a pill is far easier than sitting down for however long trying to control your thoughts. For starters, there is no waking up early involved.

4. **Meditation changes the structure of the brain**

Research by Harvard University in 2011 showed that it reduced the volume of the amygdala, the part of the brain that is responsible for fear, anxiety and stress.

When we are in the second part of the luteal phase of our cycle, when cortisol levels are increasing and we feel our anxiety levels rising, we should aim to increase our meditation levels. This is the time when we need it the most.

Incidentally, it's also the time when we can go deeper into meditation as well, as we are in a far more reflective mood and our biology is helping.

5. **Improves concentration and memory**

I discussed thought control in Chapter 10. Meditation is at

the centre of it. It involves taking hold of your monkey mind and stopping it running riot. That is bound to help with your concentration. If only this was made part of the school curriculum like PE; we would then have mental fitness as well as physical fitness. I am optimistic, though, as some schools are beginning to introduce it.

6. Meditation helps with addiction

A randomised clinical trial in the US in 2011 looked at a group of nicotine-dependent adults who smoked an average of 20 cigarettes a day. Half the group used mindfulness as a tool to help them give up, while the other half used the American Lung Association's Freedom From Smoking (FFS) treatment. At the end of the trial, the abstinence rate was 35% among those who'd practised mindfulness and 15% among those who'd used the FFS treatment. The mindfulness success rate was more than twice that of the FFS treatment. At the 17-week follow up, the gap had widened even more, with mindfulness at 31% and FFS at 6%. Mindfulness was, therefore, five times more effective.

More on meditation

Meditation to me is getting yourself to a relaxed state of mind so that you can start accessing the universal wisdom that allows you to live your best life. These days, a lot of people claim to meditate. What they really mean is that they sit down for around 10 to 15 minutes every day and try to ignore their thoughts. This is a good start and it certainly helps to calm the mind. The problem is, most of us are up and about just as our thoughts start settling down. We meditate just for a bit for breathing space and to stop us from feeling harried. We do it because it has become the new badge of honour. Within the liberal classes, spirituality is the new moral accessory.

I have been meditating for years and have tried many different styles. Even before I started doing it properly, I loved the idea of doing something calming that would set me up for the day. For years I meditated in the bath. I love a bath and had no problems getting up early to have one, so I tried to kill two birds with one stone. Things are somewhat different now, but it was a good start to help me build the habit.

There are different types of meditation techniques out there and you will have to find the one that works for you. It doesn't matter where you start, just start. Mindfulness techniques seem to have entered the zeitgeist and are being taught in the corporate world alongside other personal development courses. The bottom line is that you have to do something that calms the noisy chatter in your mind and gives you room to see the wood for the trees.

I used to think that I could go and sit cross-legged and crossed-eyed in a corner and stare at my third eye for a bit. Then chant something or other in Sanskrit (oh no, English will definitely not do, not spiritual enough, it had to be something I couldn't pronounce and couldn't possibly understand) and hey presto, I would know the answers to all the questions in the world! I would also, as a result, be calm all the time and have that sage, distant look in my eyes, exuding peace and harmony. That's me, high expectations all round!

Do you remember when we were talking about controlling your thoughts? Well, when you start meditating, and start watching your thoughts, it will quickly become apparent how much crap you think about. The mind is a tool that we have been given to help us navigate this physical dimension, but we allow it to quite literally push us all over the place. We don't assert our will with the mind because we don't know any better. It becomes the tail wagging the dog.

It's quite funny how the mind does the ecommerce thing that you get on Amazon. It goes something like this:

'People who bought this also bought that.' And then you're provided with a list.

The mind's equivalent is:

'The last time this happened, this is what you thought about, so I am going to bring it up again.'

When we are trying to buy a book on Amazon and get the 'People who bought this also bought...' we don't automatically go and buy all those things, but when the mind does it to us, we are helpless. We just buy into it and before we know it, we are in a downward spiral.

When you start to meditate, for some of you it will be your first opportunity to objectively watch your thoughts to try and observe these patterns. Then you'll start realising that just because something is in your mind does not mean that it is true or you should act on it. Sometimes it's just history. Sometimes it's the mind having nothing better to do because you have not taken control of it or given it any direction.

Just seeing the randomness of your thoughts should be enough to give you the impetus to start controlling them. This can be brought about during day-to-day meditation. So when someone comes and pushes your buttons and the mind serves up a plethora of options, most of them crap, you can take a step back and choose the option that suits you best. You don't have to be reactive. You have a choice. However, this is easier said than done.

I need to stress here that if you are not looking after yourself physically and your body is in pain, it will be nigh on impossible to sit still and meditate. If you are sleep deprived and you sit down to meditate, you will fall asleep. If you are too tired, the same thing will happen. Believe it or not, proper meditation requires a level of fitness and mental alertness. To get the best out of meditation, you need to take care of yourself.

Back to controlling the mind. For a long time, I didn't realise I had a choice in these matters. When I was triggered, that was me off for the day. The worst thing was that sometimes I would have a lovely meditation, come out of it to face the day and fall at the first hurdle. I would watch my thoughts detachedly in meditation, but that didn't translate into life. I didn't manage my thoughts when I was out of meditation. I had to work at this for years and I'm still at it. The difference now is that I am aware I have a choice. I know when my mind's ecommerce kicks in.

Many times I have come out of a meditation more wound up than when I went into it because a thought came up and rather than watch it sail on past, I had to get involved and put the world to rights. I would be the one coming out of a meditation tutting. I was getting to know myself alright, but the attitude of the said self left a lot to be desired.

You will be pleased to know that I don't come out of meditation making tutting noises anymore. I have specific types of meditation that I do when I am wound up. I am still working on the sage look in my eyes, though, but the Himalayas did not happen in a day.

Like everything, meditation is a journey and you get out of it what you put in. If you don't make the effort to manage your thoughts in meditation, it is not going to be fruitful. However, if you master the technique, it will serve you in your daily life as well. Then, when you really get established, you'll suddenly realise the power you have over your thoughts, your emotions and your world.

Do you remember how in Chapter 4 I said I wanted to tackle Maslow's hierarchy upside down?

Here is why. I believe that if you control your thoughts and emotions and let them be guided by your higher self, you will live a life that is aligned with your purpose. Once you have that clarity, the bits at the bottom of Maslow's pyramid take care of themselves. Your spirituality sets the template for your life, which influences the choices you make.

But, and here is a big but, no one is thinking of their higher self when they are hungry, feeling threatened or are unwell. Well, not us mere mortals anyway. I don't know if you have tried meditating when you are hungry. All I can think about then is pizza, and I am lactose intolerant and don't ordinarily eat it. The monkey mind takes control and causes you to crave things you can't even eat.

The fact remains that we have to take care of certain basic essentials like food, shelter and safety before we can even begin to allow ourselves to think of the 'non-essentials' like meditating. I can't believe I just wrote that because once you get to understand the importance of meditation, you will have the same attitude to it as brushing your teeth. It is part of your personal hygiene, but it just happens to be spiritual too. It sets you up for the day spiritually, mentally, emotionally and physically. Unfortunately, this is something you will have to discover for yourself.

Allow me to take you back to Chapter 4 again, when I mentioned Maslow's hierarchy and the chakras. This is where they are all going to come together nicely. Thanks for sticking with me thus far. I really couldn't wait to get here, but, like all good things in life, you have to do some grafting and kiss some frogs.

As you meditate more, you'll start to build the ability to deal with the different issues of the chakras. There are seven chakras (energy centres) in the body, starting at the base of the spine and running to the top of the head. Below is a rough guide to what is happening with each chakra:

	Chakra	Emotion	Rights
1	Root	Fear	The right to be here
2	Sacral	Guilt	The right to feel
3	Navel	Shame	The right to act
4	Heart	Grief	The right to love and be loved
5	Throat	Truth	The right to speak and hear truth
6	Third Eye	Illusion	The right to see
7	Crown	Attachment	The right to know

Table 5. Chakra Table

The parallels I draw with Maslow's pyramid are that at the base of the pyramid and at the root chakra, we are dealing with the matter of basic needs being met. That is when we are at our most fearful. As we develop and move up the chakras, other issues become more pertinent until we reach the top, which Maslow calls self-actualisation.

Spiritually speaking, this is where you have realised or got to know your higher self and your decisions are made from this place rather than from a root chakra of fear. We should all strive for that level of self-actualisation. That is where happiness resides. That is when we live a life of purpose and prioritise emotional wellbeing, physical health and personal relationships over income.

In Chapter 9, I used the LSE study and the figures to explain what contributes the most to our happiness. When you invest in meditation, you don't need research to prove this to you. You start choosing to live that way. All the data and research in the world cannot match something you have experienced for yourself, something that you know in your soul because you have tested it and it is now part of your emotional DNA.

I have this vision of me as a robot. I wake up, go and sit on my meditation mat and plug myself into my power source (the Higher Self, Divine Consciousness, whatever you are calling yours) and charge myself up to take on the day. Without that charge, I will lose power and start malfunctioning. This malfunction will not involve me falling over or anything dramatic like that, but rather it will take the form of:

- Being unable to summon the energy to exercise.
- Allowing a colleague to get to me.
- Being overwhelmed with things I normally take in my stride.
- Allowing my mind to run amok and feed me paranoia.
- Thinking the M25 motorway was built just to ruin my life. (Seriously, how self-absorbed is that? Who even knew of my existence when the M25 was being built?)
- My hair developing a mind of its own and not allowing itself to

be coerced in any way, shape or form in any direction that does not make me look like an alien.

- Feeling that the tops of my legs have ballooned overnight and I have suddenly developed thunder thighs.

Anyway, the list goes on. You literally go from having perspective to being so embroiled in the drama, you forget your gender, never mind trying to sort out follicular and luteal cycles!

You may wonder why I go on about meditation rather than the other things that people do spiritually, such as praying, reading religious text and having a quiet time in the morning. There are several ways to skin a cat but I am sure some are more efficient than others.

By all means do those things as well, but I single out meditation because it is experiential and when done correctly, it eventually changes your psychological makeup. I like meditation because it is scientific. You are changing your brain and reducing the amygdala, and therefore you are reducing fear. You are tapping into your best self by quietening your monkey mind. It puts the power in your hands.

In fact, when you start realising that you have power over your thoughts, this in itself will make you realise that the power is within you. Your higher self is within you and you just have to stop for long enough to realise this. When that happens, you'll start to make the time to meditate and feel your power. As time goes on, the quality of your meditations will improve. You'll start to enjoy the peace you'll feel when you have calmed down your thoughts. This can take years by the way, but it only takes a commitment of five minutes a day to get started.

As busy women, the demands on our time can be overwhelming, not to mention the guilt we experience when we dare to spend time on our own. There are a million and one things to do first thing in the morning. Most people feel they don't have time to sit and watch their thoughts go by in their mind. When they start meditating, some people use the time to sort out the colour of the wallpaper for the upcoming decorating or to mentally compile their shopping list. I have been there and done that. Believe it or not, I used to come up with recipes. If you think about it, when else are you going to get time to have a good ponder? These days, social media, listening to the radio and watching TV absorbs our dead time. It took me a long time to realise that meditation time was not the occasion for me to work out my issues and do my thinking. It is the exact opposite – it is for non-thinking.

If you have tried not to think before, you will know how hard it is. That is why you just have to let the mind do its thing. As long as you don't jump in and start putting the world to rights, it will gradually begin to calm down. With experience, you won't just wait for your thoughts to calm down (you haven't got all day, you know). Instead, you will take control and manage them.

This is where chanting is useful. The mind has to be given something to do to distract itself. Give it a statement of truth to focus on and by repeating it over and over again, eventually the chatter will die down and you can begin to turn your attention inward. The point of meditation is not to solve the world's problems, come up with answers or indeed acquire a sage look in your eyes. The point of meditation is to learn to 'be' so that inner wisdom can unfold. Calm your mind, tap into your higher self and then just be. By doing this, you'll allow all sorts of things to take place. Your breath will calm down completely, your heart rate will go down, there will be no disruptive thoughts to cause any disturbance, your body will be in its most relaxed state and your life force will flow easily to where it needs to be, healing what needs healing. Think about it. Every time you meditate, you allow your body to heal itself.

There are many different meditation techniques out there. Try different ones and discover the ones you get on with. Then, when you find the one that works for you, stick with it and try and go deeper. Don't keep jumping from one method to another, otherwise you will never get to go deep enough to really reap the rewards.

Let me leave you with the findings of a recent study published in 2017, which was conducted by several universities internationally. They analysed the effect of mind body interventions like yoga, meditation, tai chi, mindfulness, etc.

Their conclusion: Meditation and other mind body interventions affect your biology positively and can undo the damage caused by stress.

In Chapter 11, we reviewed stress and the negative effects of it, so here is something that reverses it. I simply love science and the direction it is going in these days. For example, quantum physics blows my mind. Scientists have started to discover what the Rishis of India have been saying for ages. No one wants to listen to a doddery old man in the Himalayas going on about how we are all matter and how different forms of matter are just energy vibrating at different frequencies. When science starts validating these things with empirical evidence, we can't continue to ignore it.

Richard Dawkins, author of *The God Delusion*, has got a book out called *Science in the Soul*. Now, Richard Dawkins is a hard-nosed scientist, so for him to even consider using the word soul in this book title is amazing. I heard him being interviewed on BBC Radio 4 and I choked up when he said science was spiritual.

To me, spirituality is the evolution of your consciousness. Meditation is an aid to that evolution. It takes the power from a bearded old man in the clouds somewhere and places it squarely in your hands. You are the point of power. The more spiritual you are, the more you grow into your power and accept the responsibility for your life. You manage your emotional wellbeing, which impacts on your children and, therefore, the next generation's wellbeing. We must not forget the impact on your partner's wellbeing either. If the world is made up of families in whatever shape or form and the primary carers – predominantly women – are finding and accepting their power through spirituality, then surely the world will be a better place.

I really could go on about this stuff, but perhaps that is another book!

PART THREE

TAKE THE BULL BY THE HORNS

CHAPTER FIFTEEN

BRINGING IT ALL TOGETHER

Before enlightenment; chop wood, carry water.
After enlightenment; chop wood, carry water.

~ ZEN PROVERB

I threw a lot at you in the previous chapters and you might be wondering how to find the time to fit it all in. Wonder no more. It can be done. I live this way. I tweak things every now and then when I find something new. It is quite easy to fit it all in once you make up your mind that this is the way you are going to live and that you are not going to do the back to front thing anymore. You are going to live according to your values and be true to yourself. Before that, though, let's talk about habits.

Habits

Your life is made up of the moments in the days, and it is what you do in those moments that count. Every little helps. You have to start with the little – your habits. What you do, day in, day out, without even thinking. Your habits compel you to do things without giving them a second thought. They make you think you like or dislike something simply because it is habit. It's now time to create new habits that are aligned with the new woman you want to become, and then repeat those habits daily.

Let me tell you something about habits and how they control us, then, hopefully, you will understand why you need new ones. As women and primary carers, this will hit home.

I once heard Nick Davies, a professor of *Behavioural Ecology*, talking on a radio programme called *The Life Scientific.* He described how a type of bird, the reed warbler, can be tricked into feeding a cuckoo chick after said chick has literally pushed the warbler's own ones out of the nest.

Apparently, the cuckoo chick sounds like a brood of warbler chicks, so the warbler gets tricked into feeding the wrong bird. This gets even more disturbing when you realise that the cuckoo chick is seven times the size of warbler chicks. There are other physical differences as well:

- The cuckoo's skin is pink while the warbler's is black.
- The cuckoo's gape is orange while the warbler's is yellow.
- The cuckoo has spots on its tongue, the warbler doesn't.

Do I hear you ask how such a mistake could be possible? Habits! They can let you do what is blatantly not serving you. In the case of the reed warbler, you feed the killer of your children. You respond to stimulus that is not correct and you don't question it because you have always done things a certain way. You are literally held hostage by your habits.

Hopefully, I have got your attention now and you will be on board with me about creating new habits so you don't end up feeding the wrong chick while yours dies! Yes, I hear you say, 'But we are not birds and we have bigger brains!' Quite right, but you get the point. Your habits can hold you hostage.

What good habits should you be incorporating into your life? Let us revise some of the things from the previous chapters. You have to be doing something in all areas of your life as an everyday habit.

- Physical: Exercise, sleep, nutrition, hydration.

- Emotional: Manage your thoughts, manage your relationships, manage your stress.
- Mental: Learn new skills, read good books.
- Spiritual: Meditate, meditate, meditate and then meditate some more.

Am I practising what I preach? Yes, for 95% of the time. Life gets in the way sometimes, but that is just life. But, as soon as it is possible, I come back to base. It is a habit so I am forced back.

What does a typical day look like?

I wake up at 6am every day, including weekends and holidays. (I have toyed with the 5am wake up several times, but I've found I'm more consistent with 6am. Maybe one day, when I get more enlightened, I will be doing the 5am thing, but for now, suffice to say, 6am works for me.)

Hydration: I drink a lemon and water tonic that my husband prepares for me (see how I get him involved?) the night before. It's 475ml, almost a quarter of my daily target of two litres. I sometimes just switch this to herbal tea. Some people drink up to a litre or more first thing, if that is you, please don't let me stop you.

Exercise: I do yoga for 20 minutes. There is nothing hard-core about this, and it isn't a particular brand of yoga you haven't heard of yet. Just my yoga for wimps – I am not leaping about in power poses, I simply do gentle stretches with breathing to release tension and energise and balance the life force in my body, in preparation for meditation.

Spiritual: Meditate for 30-40 minutes. I meditate for longer at weekends.

Exercise: Walk the dogs. We do three miles, which takes 30 minutes. I walk, speed walk or jog, depending on where I am in my cycle. At weekends we go for a longer walk because I just love walking and we could be gone for an hour to an hour and a half.

Hobby: Water the plants. This is hopefully going to be automated soon, so I will save 20 minutes in the mornings, but I must say I will miss it. I am new to gardening so I love seeing how plants change with the weather. There is something very satisfying about watching a plant grow, especially if you have planted it yourself.

Shower and get dressed. Breakfast is normally a smoothie with organic fruit, vegetables, nuts and any weird thing that I have read is good for me. No one is going to make me a smoothie with all the weird stuff that I normally put in mine, so I cut out the middleman and make it myself. It only takes me seven minutes. Yes, I have timed it.

When I am really tight on time and can't make a smoothie, I make Nutella (this is so decadent yet my recipe is so healthy, it takes me a minute, probably the same time it would take me to spread the shop-bought additives-packed version) and have it with homemade, wholemeal soda bread. I sometimes run weekend residential workshops about how to put it all together and we bake the soda bread and make the Nutella just to demonstrate how easy it is to eat well.

I take two pieces of fruit to work with me. At the weekend, I tend to have a cooked breakfast with my family at the table or we go out for breakfast. A cooked breakfast for us is assorted roast vegetables, eggs, salmon and brown bread.

I will normally hit my recommended five a day fruit and vegetable intake just eating breakfast alone. After that, even if I get completely derailed and have to eat rubbish, at least I know I had a decent start.

If I am in my bleeding phase, I will think nothing of asking for breakfast in bed at the weekend. It's not because I am ill or there is something wrong with me, it's because I am worth it and deserve to take time out to rejuvenate. One weekend out of four is not too much to ask. I am happy to cook breakfast for everyone at weekends because I love cooking, but I am just as happy to be waited on.

As I've said before, I used to be one of those people who was 'too busy' to have breakfast. These days I know better, so I make the time. Apart from the fact that I don't want any blood sugar spikes and crashes, I also don't want to get myself so hungry that I eat rubbish before lunch.

By the time I head out of the door, I have done my Spiritual, I have done my Exercise and I have made a decent stab at Hydration and Nutrition. I am all set to roll with the punches of the day.

I normally have an hour's commute to the office, but this is subject to the vagaries of the M25 and it can sometimes take an hour and a half. This is a godsend. An hour to an hour and a half to myself with no interruptions! If you are a mother, you'll know how rare that is. (One of my sons sometimes calls out my name, just so he can get it out of his head he says. I constantly hear 'Mum, Mum, Mum' and feel I am always on call.)

I top up on my Mental by listening to good programmes, audiobooks, podcasts and CDs, etc., in the car. I reckon I do the equivalent of a degree every year just on my drive to and from work. I can also sometimes be found singing and dancing behind the wheel. I am one of those people who can't listen to a good song without singing along. If it requires movement, well, I can manage that while keeping my hands on the wheel. I am sure the police would have a thing or two to say about such behaviour.

I used to bring my lunch to the office, but some person in health and safety decided that grownups can't be allowed to heat up food in the microwave. So now there are no microwaves. This leaves me with the office canteen food. I don't work for Google where they have rock star chefs. The chefs at my workplace have stars in their eyes alright, but for reasons I dare not venture into.

The food is so bland that I can spend a lot of time at the condiment counter looking for a way to spice it up. I will normally have a jacket potato with a tuna or mackerel salad, or an Asian broth with vegetables and prawns. Thursday is curry day. I explained earlier how I turn this into a healthy version.

Relationships: Whenever I can, I arrange a lunch date, as social interactions are good for one's soul. I rarely sit with colleagues and let lunch become an extension of work. I prefer to make the effort to invite people for one-on-one lunches. I love chatting. This normally happens in the third week of my cycle when I am in the summer of my phase and feel like the life and soul.

Office relationships can be quite superficial so I value these one-on-one chats, where people open up more. You suddenly get a window into a female colleague's life and can offer a kind word or a listening ear over a jacket potato. Women don't want to bore the men at work with their childcare issues. In a perfect world, they would be just as interested, but we all know this isn't the case.

In the fourth week of my cycle, I can sometimes be found lunching alone. This is the autumn of my cycle, when I am more reflective. Sometimes I don't want a lot of people in my space. I am just as happy to grab a quick lunch and then go for a solitary walk.

Dinner is normally protein, mainly fish and organic vegetables; salads in the summer, soups in the winter.

I spent years fighting the organic food movement in my head and thinking of it as a waste of money. I don't think that anymore, but this book is not long enough for me to go into the ins and outs. I believe I have laid out my eating philosophy in a previous chapter. I tend to stay away from starchy carbohydrates in the evenings.

Social: I try to meet one girlfriend for dinner and a catch up on life once a month, but this can be challenging. People are so busy and these days you have to book these things a million years in advance.

Whenever the weather is nice, at weekends, I try to drag people over for a barbeque. I suppose in the UK we can never take the weather for granted. I am quite a good cook so people will normally say yes to an invite. That said, nobody is ever that fussed about barbeque food, as it's generally accepted that it will comprise burnt burgers and undercooked meats, so anything other than this is considered a triumph. My barbeques tend to be made up of whole foods and tonnes of fish, and I do cave in and cook some good-quality sausages or steak burgers for the kids. I am a party animal and never say no to a party if I can help it. I don't always have to have people over to have a barbeque. If the weather is nice then dinner is cooked outside. When everyone else but me is fed up of eating al fresco, I have been known to put a solitary mackerel on the barbeque.

If all this sounds a bit like *The Good Life* in the suburbs and a tad overwhelming, as mentioned earlier, I run weekend residential workshops in small, intimate groups where I show people how to put this all together. It is a nurturing environment where we go through the physical, emotional, mental and spiritual. I guess it is a bit like a grownup pyjama party, only you learn life skills to help you live authentically.

When I say I live this stuff, I mean it. It is my lifestyle. The workshops started when I invited a friend over for brunch. I threw something together casually, which took me all of 30 minutes, but she was amazed. She couldn't believe how most of what we had eaten was homemade, organic and seemed to have been rustled up with the minimum of effort.

'I'd eat like that if I knew what to do,' she said.

You have to believe me when I say it doesn't take a lot. You just have to make the decision to prioritise your health and eat well. You need a few basics and then you will be surprised how creative you can get.

For example, for a dinner of barbequed mackerel accompanied by a spinach and tomato salad with French mustard dressing, the only processed part of the meal will be the mustard, as this will come from a jar. Everything else is just mixing stuff and putting fish on the barbeque, which takes 20 minutes to cook. So this delicious, good looking and wholesome meal can be rustled up in 30 minutes max, and that includes making a salad dressing from scratch.

We have looked at waking up, breakfast and then lunch through to dinner. What next? Whatever you do to relax in the evening is up to you, but between dinner and homework, there isn't normally that much time left, apart from maybe an hour for TV if I am lucky. I don't watch anything past 10pm, as this is when I head upstairs to get ready for bed.

My bedroom is my sanctuary. No TV is allowed and I put my phone on silent. Depending on where I am in my cycle, I might take longer to get ready for bed. If it is a weekday, then it is the usual hygiene stuff, then read something spiritual, take a mantra or affirmation, and repeat it to myself until I fall asleep.

If I am in self-care mode, then I will come up a bit earlier and have a luxurious bath. This will normally be at weekends when I have a bit more time. Also, in the autumn of my cycle, when I am feeling reflective, I will think nothing of cutting out TV and retiring to bed early to read or write.

There you go. You can pack it all in, but it is the day-to-day that matters; what you do day in, day out, rather than the odd dinner with a friend. You have to build habits to sustain you. Decide what you want and build habits around this. Before you know it, you will be living the life of your dreams, feeling healthy and looking good on it.

CHAPTER SIXTEEN

THE LIFE THAT LOOKS GOOD ON YOU

There is no enlightenment outside of daily life.

~ THICH NHAT HANH

I started off by saying how we live our lives back to front and how we are always stressed out as a result. Hopefully, I have taken you through enough things to make you want to make changes that work for you. It can be done. It doesn't matter where you are coming from or what you have done or haven't done in the past. You can build your perfect life one day at a time through your new habits.

I have this vision that one day women will realise how beautifully complicated they are and how without them society wouldn't function.

The gender ratio in most species is approximately 1:1. In humans, for every 107 boys, 100 girls are born. We form half the population but our influence way outstrips this 50% ratio. We are the lynchpin of society. I once read an article in *The New Scientist* that argued that educating girls could combat global warming. Go figure! Well, the link was not as tenuous as you might think. The argument, which I haven't got space to go into here, was sheer elegance. Basically, the more educated a woman is, the less likely she is to have a big family. This will help to control population growth and because global warming is significantly affected by human activity and population, educating women is good for the planet. (Suffice to say, ladies, even saving the environment is hinged on us.)

Unfortunately, the very important role that women play is what sometimes imprisons them. We feel obliged to make sacrifices that we later grow to resent. All my life I knew I had to write, but my life was just not set up to support a writer's lifestyle. I didn't quite buy into the romantic notion of being a struggling artist. From my early 20s, I had financial responsibilities and I never felt I had the freedom to do what made my heart sing. It was duty before pleasure.

So, I embarked on the treacherous greasy pole, which is the corporate ladder. I knew no different, and the people I looked up to had chosen that route too. Society places a lot of value on ostentatious material trinkets and some of us find our self-worth wrongfully tied up in these said trinkets. This continues until our body stages a coup and our hormones hold us hostage because we have lived a life of imbalance for so long. I wouldn't mind it if we did that as women and got the recognition we deserve. Still, I shall not be bitter! Those of us still working on the sage look in our eyes know the futility of this.

I am always astounded that in this day and age women still have to fight for recognition. It makes my mind boggle that women are still held back from the higher echelons of the church and have to fight for their place in parliament and in corporate boardrooms. Surely we all know enough to know that it is women who make the world go round?

Maybe it is clear for me to see because I am a woman and a descendent of Yaa Asantewaa, the warrior queen of the Ashanti Kingdom in Ghana. She was my great-great grandmother. According to legend, at the beginning of 1900, as well as arming herself and her women to fight the British, Yaa Asantewaa also inspired them to use 'biological' warfare to make their husbands launch a siege on the fort that the British were using as a refuge against a local rebellion. The 'biological' warfare by the women was a pledge not to sleep with their husbands until the British had been capitulated. All's fair in love and war, right?

Growing up with such a rich heritage of strong women who had the same rights as men, you can see why I'm confounded by the fact that more than a century on, women have to fight for their place at the table. It is almost like we've taken a backward step.

Around the world now, there are still matrilineal and matriarchal societies, so all is not lost. A few examples are:

- The Musuo, located near the borders of Tibet
- The Minangkabau of West Sumatra, near Tibet
- The Akan in Ghana, West Africa
- The Talamanca in Costa Rica
- The Khasi and the Garos of North East India

These tribes have women actively involved in governance and politics, child rearing, spiritual matters, business and commerce. Women are seen as equal, although some tasks are still seen as female roles, typically aligned with their strengths and biology.

Professor Schuller, in his book *The Paula Principle*, argues that most women work below their level of competence. He points out that 40-45% of women work part-time and unless the attitude towards part-time work changes, women will never shatter the glass ceiling. There might be the odd poke through it, but you'd need a critical mass for it to permeate the mass consciousness.

Let's have a look at why a lot of women choose to work part-time. Is it because of our caring duties? Why should society penalise us for choosing to bring up the next generation or caring for our elderly, who made our generation possible? Shouldn't women be applauded for making decisions like this? They say you can tell a lot about a society by how it treats its vulnerable. I will stretch this to say you can tell a lot about a society by how its treats those who look after its vulnerable.

As mentioned in an earlier chapter, I had the temerity to get pregnant while working and, before I could say nappy rash, I had been made redundant. Now, why should a lactating mother be one of the first to go when an organisation is restructuring? The fact that I brought in a multitude of skills gained from my education and experience and could get up in the morning, feed a baby, express milk for when I was out of the office, sort out a nanny, sort out dinner and still be in the office at the same time as my male colleagues, who'd just rolled out of bed, was neither here nor there. My multi-tasking and ability to spin eight plates at the same time somehow got discounted simply because I was lactating. Give me a break!

Women are pivotal to society. We have to make sure we are valued for what we bring to the party. To do this we have to value and take care of ourselves. We are still fighting a few battles on several fronts to get the recognition that we deserve and until that happens, and I am optimistic enough to believe equal opportunities will happen, we owe it to ourselves to live our best lives.

That life should not be back to front. You need to set your lens, your template, whatever you choose to call it, and that lens should be set by your values. Your values should be what brings you joy and aligns you with your purpose. What do you think you were put on this earth for? What makes your heart sing? What does a good life look like to you? List all the elements you would like in your life then test to see if they are aligned with your values. If you don't do this test, you will forever be fighting an uphill battle. If you don't value good health (and I can't for the life of me think why anyone wouldn't) then you will find it difficult to get your behind up in the morning to exercise. If you don't value family and close personal relationships and therefore haven't scheduled them into your life, then you are climbing the wrong ladder.

For those of you thinking, 'What are my values?' They should cover:

- Physical
- Mental

- Emotional
- Spiritual

Don't leave any of them out.

Allow me to fantasise here. In my view, here is someone living their best life:

- They look good
- They feel good
- They eat well
- They have somehow managed to find out how to do what they love for a living and make a decent living out of it
- They have friends
- They know how to conduct difficult conversations and they don't shy away from them
- They understand the importance of family
- They have a hobby that they thoroughly enjoy
- They are financially responsible
- They contribute to their society in whatever way they deem fit
- They have a twinkle in their eye and understand how to squeeze every ounce out of life
- They have a positive outlook
- They value themselves enough to carve out time every day for meditation and/or contemplation
- They see people for who they are rather than for what they have

This is not an exhaustive list by the way. Feel free to add your own.

Do you know anyone like that? If not, you are about to become that person.

If you take the things we have discussed in this book on board, your life will be transformed. It doesn't matter where you start, you could just begin with eating well. The other things will soon follow. If you asked me where to start, though, I would say meditation. Carve out that time for yourself every day to be with your higher self. You are worth it. It doesn't matter what type of meditation you do, just do it. Don't let your day be highjacked before you have even had a chance to start. Take that time for yourself.

We live in a quick-fix culture, where everything is instant and no one wants to wait for anything anymore. But to take on board the suggestions in this book is a lifestyle choice. It is not a quick fix, although you will start to see changes in your body and energy levels within a couple of weeks of eating and sleeping well.

You owe it to yourself to embark on this journey and live the life that suits you. You also owe it to your children, your family and your animals. Just by virtue of being a woman and a mother means you are holding a lot of people up. You cannot afford to continue like an Octopus on a Treadmill flailing around all the time. It is not efficient. You will wear yourself out. You will find yourself one day looking a doctor in the eye and trying to process some news that could have been prevented given half a chance. You don't want to be tracking 14 symptoms on a spreadsheet and going from doctor to doctor.

Life is an adventure. For a long time I was always afraid. Fear became a habit until I wasn't even sure what I was afraid of anymore. My physical and medical challenges also added to this fear. I was constantly battling a roller coaster of emotions. I was hurtling towards an early menopause at the rate of knots. I decided there was another way to live life.

I didn't want to live in fear anymore. I wanted to look life squarely in the eye and say 'bring it on'. It has been a long journey but I can honestly say, hand on heart, that I made all the changes that I recommend in this book. I am a different woman now and the fact that I even have the balls to write this book is a testament to that.

Our lives are complex. We all have our challenges to face, but rather than facing life from a deficit and being reliant on caffeine and prescription drugs to power us through while feeling semi-detached from our reality, we know enough now to take care of ourselves. We therefore have a fighting chance of bringing out the best in ourselves in the way we are designed to be. It's exquisite!

I am

I am woman, I am complex,
I am woman, I am free.

I can live and learn to live the life,
That I deserve to see.

I am woman, I am elemental,
I am woman, I long to be.

All that every woman dreams,
To be, to be supreme.

Gifty Enright

ACKNOWLEDGEMENTS

I am very grateful to Andrew Hill for allowing me to use his story.

To my friends Geanie Asante, Kate Golding and Tin Gill, for encouraging me to keep going and not allowing me to wimp out.

To Laura Thornhill, my PA, for being the woman behind the woman. Thank you for being four of my eight tentacles. To my cousin, Brandie Deignan, for phoning me on the M25 most mornings to ensure that I was still sane.

To my ever-supportive husband, David, and my kids, Tadg and Finn, for their patience and for putting up with me locking myself away in the study for hours on end.

A NOTE FROM GIFTY

Thank you for taking the time to read *Octopus on a Treadmill*. I hope you enjoyed it and that the information and advice will help you to improve your work-life balance.

Do you want more?

Sign up to my blog to continue the journey and be notified of any pending book releases or updated content.

What are you waiting for?

Sign up now: **www.giftyenright.com/blog/**

You can also join my closed facebook group to continue the conversation with other like- minded women. Here is the link: www.facebook.com/groups/octopusseries/

If you would like to find out more about my work, please visit my website: www.giftyenright.com

Thank you so much for choosing to go on this journey with me. I am glad that you stopped by.

Please do not hesitate to connect with me if you have any questions about this book, or if you just want someone to chat with.

I would be happy to hear from you and I enjoy connecting with readers.

Thanks again,

Gifty Enright

YOUR FREE RESOURCE

In addition to the information already provided in this book, I have created a Life Map Tracker that will help you track your progress in the different areas of your life.

To receive your free bonus Life Map Tracker, sign up for my mailing list by visiting: **www.giftyenright.com/a-life-map/**

Signing up will also notify you of any pending book releases or updated content. By subscribing, you will be first in line for exclusive deals and future book giveaways.

Immediately after signing up, you will be given access to download the Life Map Tracker.

Gifty Enright

A QUICK FAVOUR, PLEASE?

Before you go, can I ask you for a quick favour?

Good, I knew I could count on you.

Would you please leave this book a review on Amazon?

Reviews are very important for authors, as they help us sell more books. This will in turn enable me to write more books for you.

Please take a quick minute to go to Amazon and leave this book an honest review. I promise it doesn't take very long, but it will help this book reach more readers just like you.

Thank you for reading, and thank you so much for being part of the journey.

Gifty Enright

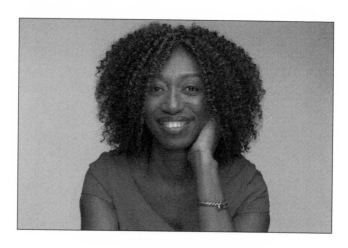

About the Author

Alongside her work as an author, Gifty Enright provides consulting services to multinational companies on major transformation programmes. She is also the Managing Director of a sports events company.

Gifty has travelled extensively throughout Europe, the Americas and across Asia. She has spent the last twenty years studying the hectic life of the busy working mother and the effects it has on women and their health (physical, emotional and spiritual). Her book *Octopus on a Treadmill* is based on her lifelong experience across diverse cultures, research and science. It is about how to maintain balance and not lose yourself, while spinning all the plates as a working mother.

Born in Kumasi, the ancient capital of the Ashanti people in Ghana, Gifty has lived for the past thirty years in Hertfordshire in the UK. She is married with two children.

Gifty marries the science of the West, Eastern philosophy and the wisdom of Africa; like you, dear reader, Gifty is a female explorer. She hopes you will enjoy this new adventure.

To find out more about Gifty's work, please see her website **www.giftyenright.com.**

Made in the USA
Columbia, SC
08 January 2019